Couples, Trauma, and Catastrophes

Couples, Trauma, and Catastrophes has been co-published simultaneously as *Journal of Couples Therapy*, Volume 7, Number 4 1998.

Couples, Trauma, and Catastrophes

Barbara Jo Brothers
Editor

Couples, Trauma, and Catastrophes has been co-published simultaneously as *Journal of Couples Therapy*, Volume 7, Number 4 1998.

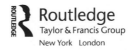

Routledge
Taylor & Francis Group
New York   London

Couples, Trauma, and Catastrophes has been co-published simultaneously as *Journal of Couples Therapy,* Volume 7, Number 4 1998.

© 1998 by The Haworth Press, Inc. All rights reserved. No part of this work may be reproduced or utilized in any form or by any means, electronic or mechanical, including photocopying, microfilm and recording, or by any information storage and retrieval system, without permission in writing from the publisher.

The development, preparation, and publication of this work has been undertaken with great care. However, the publisher, employees, editors, and agents of The Haworth Press and all imprints of The Haworth Press, Inc., including The Haworth Medical Press® and Pharmaceutical Products Press®, are not responsible for any errors contained herein or for consequences that may ensue from use of materials or information contained in this work. Opinions expressed by the author(s) are not necessarily those of The Haworth Press, Inc.

First published 1998 by
The Haworth Press, Inc., 10 Alice Street, Binghamton, NY 13904-1580

This edition published 2013 by Routledge
711 Third Avenue, New York, NY 10017
2 Park Square, Milton Park, Abingdon, Oxon OX14 4RN

Routledge is an imprint of the Taylor & Francis Group, an informa business

Cover design by Thomas J. Mayshock Jr.

Library of Congress Cataloging-in-Publication Data

Couples, trauma, and catastrophes/Barbara Jo Brothers, editor.
    p. cm.
    "Has been co-published simultaneously as Journal of couples therapy, Volume 7, Number 4, 1998."
    Includes bibliographical references and index.
    ISBN 0-7890-0532-8 (alk. paper).–ISBN 0-7890-0546-8 (alk. paper)
    1. Marital psychotherapy. 2. Psychic trauma. 3. Life change events. 4. Crisis intervention (Psychiatry) I. Brothers, Barbara Jo, 1940- . II. Journal of couples therapy.
RC488.5.C647 1998
616.89′ 156–dc21   98-35597
                                                                                                          CIP

Couples, Trauma, and Catastrophes

CONTENTS

ABOUT THE EDITOR

Barbara Jo Brothers, MSW, BCD, a Diplomate in Clinical Social Work, National Association of Social Workers, is in private practice in New Orleans. She received her BA from the University of Texas and her MSW from Tulane University, where she is currently on the faculty. She was Editor of *The Newsletter of the American Academy of Psychotherapists* from 1976 to 1985, and was Associate Editor of *Voices: The Art and Science of Psychotherapy* from 1979 to 1989. She has 30 years of experience, in both the public and private sectors, helping people to form skills that will enable them to connect emotionally. The author of numerous articles and book chapters on authenticity in human relating, she has advocated healthy, congruent communication that builds intimacy as opposed to destructive, incongruent communication which blocks intimacy. In addition to her many years of direct work with couples and families, Ms. Brothers has led numerous workshops on teaching communication in families and has also played an integral role in the development of training programs in family therapy for mental health workers throughout the Louisiana state mental health system. She is a board member of the Institute for International Connections, a non-profit organization for cross-cultural professional development focused on training and cross-cultural exchange with psychotherapists in Russia, republics once part of what used to be the Soviet Union, and other Eastern European countries.

Ways of Viewing the World:
"... Living Our Lives
by Somebody Else's Pattern ... "

Virginia Satir

EDITOR'S NOTE. The following excerpt was taken from Virginia Satir's lecture in 1983 which she titled "Ways of Perceiving the World," one of a series of lectures: Avanta Process Community Meeting III, Crested Butte, Colorado, August 1983. It must be understood that this edited transcription is taken out of context. The lecture was delivered during a thirty day seminar and was part of preparation for training therapists in the Satir Model. Exercises and demonstrations before and after the lectures were part of the training experience.

In this lecture, Virginia is giving one of her key insights: destructive behavior is a person's attempt to deal with the fear of inadequacy, failure, and not measuring up in the eyes of others. She begins by pointing out that children learn to define themselves through the eyes of their parents, going on to use the metaphor of the Procrustean Bed as a graphic illustration of the damage people do to themselves in trying to substitute another person's picture for their own identity.

Printed with permission of John Banmen, Delta Psychological Associates, Inc., 11213 Canyon Crescent, Delta, B.C., Canada V41 2R6. All copyrights reserved.

This lecture transcript is part of a series that appears in past and subsequent issues of the *Journal of Couples Therapy*.

[Haworth co-indexing entry note]: "Ways of Viewing the World: '.. Living Our Lives by Somebody Else's Pattern . . . '" Satir, Virginia. Co-published simultaneously in *Journal of Couples Therapy* (The Haworth Press, Inc.) Vol. 7, No. 4, 1998, pp. 1-4; and: *Couples, Trauma, and Catastrophes* (ed: Barbara Jo Brothers) The Haworth Press, Inc., 1998, pp. 1-4.

DEFINITION OF A PERSON

Now, we come to the next part. What is the definition of a person? For people who hold the threat and reward approach, the definition of a person is someone who should conform and obey. The symbol I use for that one is a box. How many of you have found yourselves saying, "I'm too much of this and I should be something of that?" Those are the "too" twins, too much of what I am and should be something else. That means I have to make myself in the way that somebody else wants. To do that means then that I have to cut myself off (Satir, 1987).

. . . [So] what I found in the definition of a person is that there was like a square–or an oblong, whatever it was–a box that I had to fit into to conform and to obey. And so my image of myself as a person was whether or not I conformed and obeyed to whatever it was that I "should." Now, "shoulds" are hierarchy from the people who were our survival figures. Whether they meant it or not, that is where it came from–"What you should be for me to love you." We have already had plenty of examples. "I should be perfect," and the rest of that is "or you won't be loved." or "I should always do it right or I won't be loved." Or "I should never talk back to my mother." Or "I should never let you know I am angry at you." All those kinds of things.

So my definition of myself depends upon living my "shoulds" which are in all innocence–you are trying to be good. And there are malevolent and benevolent forms. About four weeks before I came out here I heard about a group of people in California that were under the name of a religious group who were starting to beat the children at age 14 days so they would grow up without the devil in them. Now from where they were, you can see how much they were related to what they said was the right way to be.

PROCRUSTEAN BED

Now I am going to give you just a little bit of a metaphor to tie this to. Some of you may remember the procrustean bed. We look back . . . [to] when they tortured people–and you know that was all then, we do not do that now. But anyway, there was a procrustean bed. Now this was referred to by some people as a very successful rehabilitation instrument, and anyone who was outside of the main swing of things for whatever reason would be sent to the procrustean bed for rehabilitation. And it is true that it always succeeded, but let me tell you how. It turned out that this procrustean bed never really fit anybody, so you were always too short or too long for it. Now if you were too short they cut you in half in the middle. That is where you would be if you were in half in the middle, wouldn't you? If you were too long they cut off your head and feet. You fit the bed perfectly, treatment perfectly successful. The only problem was you were not there to enjoy it.

We are still doing stuff like that. Now let us look at it. Cut here and we cut off the solar plexus, the basis for which we can be in harmony, our feeling. "Don't you dare feel differently from me!" People have been burned for different feelings. Now let us look at feet. "Don't you dare move differently from me!" That is the risk-taking part. Now let us look at the head. "Don't you dare think differently from me!" O.K. how many of us have had thoughts, have had feelings, have had ideas, and we have said to ourselves, "I can't do it," because if we do we will encounter wrath. So we live by our "shoulds." Maybe some of you here will make a "should" song, and its called "shoulding on yourself."

Now let us look at what happens here. To take this beautiful being that we have and to shave off everything except what is exactly like you–[this] means that we are trying to live life in a way that does not fit us. It does not fit us. Now what happens when we do that? Well, we have to start squeezing and so our natural feeling of this is to feel deprived, limited and great fear because it comes back again. Fear is the greatest thing that we have to deal with, great fear. "What if I don't do it right?" You know what that means? "What if I don't do it the way somebody else wants it." That is all it means. And we are right now so completely–in relation to where it is going here–so completely living our lives by somebody else's pattern. And so we have deprivation, limitation, and great fear . . .

LIFE FORCE

Now what do human beings do when they feel deprived and limited? That has something to do with the *life-force*. And what does the life-force do? *Life-force can not be killed, it has to be reformed . . . It can be reformed into very negative behavior*, into gruesome kinds of physical anomalies and difficulties, into hatreds because the amount of energy that goes into a hatred thing is a very big one. *It's displaced energy from someone who feels deprived and knows no other way to go.* So what we begin to find here then are all the defenses we use and all the rationalizations we use for that defense.

Human beings cannot live with fear, they have to do something about it. And we come back to our old friends: to project . . . "It's your fault," to deny. . . "Oh, no it's not". . . . "Oh, I didn't see that." So we end up being nincompoops, but we're nincompoops not because we want to [be], we're nincompoops because we're trying to be good. That is what is so sad (1983, p. 206-209).

REFERENCES

Banmen, J. and Satir, V. (1983) *Virginia Satir verbatim*. John Banmen Delta Psychological Associates, Inc. 11213 Canyon Crescent, North Delta, British Columbia, Canada V4E 2R6.

Satir, V. (1987). Speaker. Avanta Process Community VII, Module I. Cassette Recordings. Crested Butte, Colorado: Blue Moon Cassettes.

The Art of Working
with Traumatized Couples

Jim Lantz
Andy Stuck

SUMMARY. In this article, the authors present a framework for treatment of the traumatized couple and also their belief in the importance of seeing such work as a process of art. Clinical illustrations are used to demonstrate their approach. *[Article copies available for a fee from The Haworth Document Delivery Service: 1-800-342-9678. E-mail address: getinfo@haworthpressinc.com]*

Working with traumatized couples (and their children) is an artistic process that blends the subjective and objective elements of treatment in a useful and meaningful way (Lantz, 1974, 1993, 1994A, 1994B). Although it is important for the couple's therapist to have a knowledge base and a treatment framework, the real work that is healing to the traumatized couple is always unique to the couple and the therapist and is generally "newly" created by the couple and therapist during the treatment process (Lantz, 1993, 1994C). Viktor Frankl (1959) makes this point through his formula T = X + Y. In Frankl's (1959) formula, T = good therapy, X = the unique treatment needs of the client and Y = the unique characteristics and

Jim Lantz, PhD, is Co-Director of Lantz and Lantz Counseling Associates and Associate Professor at The Ohio State University, College of Social Work, 1947 College Road, Columbus, OH 43210.

Andy Stuck, PhD, is Director of Day Treatment at Hannah Neil Center for Children, Columbus, OH.

[Haworth co-indexing entry note]: "The Art of Working with Traumatized Couples." Lantz, Jim, and Andy Stuck. Co-published simultaneously in *Journal of Couples Therapy* (The Haworth Press, Inc.) Vol. 7, No. 4, 1998, pp. 5-18; and: *Couples, Trauma, and Catastrophes* (ed: Barbara Jo Brothers) The Haworth Press, Inc., 1998, pp. 5-18. Single or multiple copies of this article are available for a fee from The Haworth Document Delivery Service [1-800-342-9678, 9:00 a.m. - 5:00 p.m. (EST). E-mail address: getinfo@haworthpressinc.com].

© 1998 by The Haworth Press, Inc. All rights reserved.

5

capacities of the therapist. Although such creativity and art are the hall-marks of effective treatment with traumatized couples (Lantz, 1974, 1995, 1996, in press), we believe that such artistic healing occurs most frequent-ly when the therapist actively focuses the treatment process upon helping the couple to "hold" the trauma, "tell" the trauma, "master" the trauma and "honor" the trauma (Lantz, 1974, 1993, 1995). We also believe that these four elements of treatment are most useful with couples who have been traumatized from "outside" the couple's relationship system and are not effective with couples who have been traumatized from "within" the relationship system, such as in situations of spousal abuse (Lantz, 1978). The following sections of the article will describe and illustrate the art of helping couples to hold, tell, master and honor the traumas that have impacted upon their intimate life. Figure 1 illustrates the relationship between the treatment elements of holding, telling, mastering and honor-ing and the stages of treatment with traumatized couples.

THE ART OF HOLDING THE TRAUMA

Trauma is often repressed, ignored, avoided, and pushed into the cou-ple's unconsciousness in order to avoid the experience of trauma pain. Holding the trauma is a process of "holding up" the trauma so it may be seen, remembered, and re-experienced. Unfortunately (and fortunately), holding up the trauma includes re-experiencing the pain and suffering that are always a part of the trauma experience (Lantz, 1993). Holding up the trauma includes catharsis. As the couple holds, remembers and re-experi-ences the trauma, there is generally a release of pain that frequently re-duces (but does not eliminate) the level of on-going suffering that the couple will experience (Lantz, 1974, 1993, 1995).

Helping the couple to hold the trauma requires that the couple's thera-pist also hold the couple's trauma pain and hold the traumatized couple as

FIGURE 1

Stages of Treatment	Treatment Dynamics			
	Holding	Telling	Mastering	Honoring
Initial Stage	X	X		
Middle Stage		X	X	
Ending Stage			X	X

they are remembering and re-experiencing the trauma pain (Lantz, 1974, 1993). Such holding has been described by Winnicott (1989) as providing an "adequate holding environment" and by Lindy (1988) as "walking point." We prefer to use Gabriel Marcel's (1951, 1956, 1963) concept of empathic availability to describe and understand this component of treatment.

Empathic availability (Marcel, 1956; Lantz, 1994C) is a committed presence to the "other" and an openness to the pain and potentials of the other even when such openness is difficult and unpleasant. Urban-Appalachian couples often describe availability as loyalty. It has also been described as integrity (Andrews, 1972) and as an ability to experience the pain of the other without a loss of personal identity and/or personal sense of self (Mullan and Sangiuliano, 1964).

When manifesting empathic availability, the therapist does not hide from the couple's pain behind an ardent stance of objectivity and/or abstraction nor behind a belief in an overly rigid interpretation of the treatment role (Lantz, 1994C). Although the psychotherapist who works with traumatized couples must remember to stick to the treatment role, such a concern with role should not result in "blunted" encounter and/or compassion nor be used to distance the therapist from the couple's pain. Empathic availability often provides the couple with the support needed to help them "tell" the story of their trauma experiences (Lantz, 1993). Empathic availability gives the traumatized couple a feeling of "really being understood" (Van Kaam, 1959; Lantz, 1994C, 1996).

Empathic availability is probably not occurring unless the therapist begins to experience secondary post-traumatic stress disorder symptoms (Lantz, 1974, 1993, 1995; Lindy, 1988). If a traumatized couple's therapist is really helping the couple to "hold up" the trauma pain, the therapist will begin to personally experience bits, slivers, and elements of the couple's pain (Lantz, 1974, 1978, 1993). This process is illustrated in Figure 2.

The therapist's empathic availability and willingness to hold and share the couple's trauma pain allows the couple to hold up and remember their trauma pain. In our experience, the couple is often able to remember their trauma or traumas reactive to the therapist's empathic availability, and the couple will repress and/or continue to repress their awareness of trauma without the support of the therapist's empathic availability.

THE ART OF TELLING THE TRAUMA

Telling, talking about, and naming trauma and trauma pain is the second phase and/or element of treatment with a traumatized couple. Para-

FIGURE 2

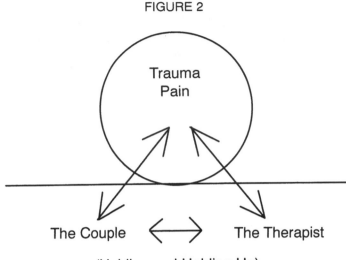

The Couple ⟷ The Therapist

(Holding and Holding Up)

doxically, telling the trauma both depends upon the development of encounter and empathic availability between therapist and couple and powerfully facilitates development of such encounter (Lantz, 1974, 1993, 1994C, 1996). Telling the trauma is helpful to the couple for two basic reasons. First, such telling is helpful as it places the trauma experience and trauma pain into the interactional world of encounter where the relationship between the couple and between the couple and the therapist can be used to help process the trauma under conditions of increased support (Andrews, 1972; Lantz, 1974, 1993). Telling the trauma brings trauma pain out of the internal, unconscious world of the traumatized couple and into the interactional world of mutual awareness, understanding, encounter, and support (Andrews, 1971; Figley, 1989; Lantz, 1974, 1995; Mullan and Sangiuliano, 1964).

A second reason why telling the trauma is helpful has to do with the power of naming. When a couple can describe, tell and name the trauma or traumas they have experienced, this is often the beginning of processing and/or mastering the trauma (Lantz, 1978). An example of such telling and naming occurred in treatment with Mr. and Mrs. Jones. Mrs. Jones was an adult survivor of childhood sexual abuse. In the fourth conjoint treatment session with Mr. and Mrs. Jones, Mrs. Jones was able to remember and tell about how the "man next door" forced her to do oral sex (i.e., oral rape) when she was a child. She also was able to remember and tell how this man would take nude photographs of her before and after the oral rape.

Mrs. Jones reported that "for years" she had become "horribly nervous" whenever anyone would try to photograph her. Mrs. Jones had always felt "nuts" about this "photo phobia" until she was able to remember and tell about her awful childhood experiences. Telling and renaming the "photo phobia" events helped Mrs. Jones to feel more "in control." In her words, she no longer felt like "a mental case." Instead, she felt "like a normal person–who the hell wouldn't have gotten afraid if this kind of shit had happened to them?"

THE ART OF MASTERING THE TRAUMA

Charles Figley (1989) reports that helping a couple to find, develop, and utilize a "healing theory" is an important way to help them master the trauma. To Figley (1989), helping a couple to discover and use a healing theory is a process of reflection and experimentation that helps each member of the couple find unique healing activities that are personally useful in processing and mastering the trauma. From our existential point of view, helping the couple to develop a healing theory means helping them to find both a meaning, reason, and/or purpose for change and also specific methods and activities of change that are compatible with their skills, abilities, and strengths (Lantz, 1974, 1994B, 1996). In our view, Frankl (1959) has presented one of the most heroic examples of how to discover a reason, meaning, and purpose for change in a traumatic situation, and Ochberg and Fojtik (1984), as well as Figley (1989), have presented important techniques that can be utilized to process and master a trauma.

THE ART OF HONORING THE TRAUMA

The art of honoring the trauma refers to the process of identifying and making use of meaning potentials and opportunities that can be found in the trauma situation. To Viktor Frankl (1959), honoring the trauma involves becoming consciously aware of some of the opportunities for self-transcendent giving to the world that are embedded in the trauma situation and in the trauma memory. In the process of honoring the trauma, the existential psychotherapist helps the couple to find and actualize a desire to give birth to another's joy and/or to facilitate the cessation of another's pain that is reactive to their empathic understanding of trauma and the trauma pain of other human beings. For example:

Bill served in combat in Vietnam in 1966 and 1967. When he came home, he married Sally, and he finished college in 1971. Bill, Jr. was born in 1970. Bill, Sr. was symptom-free for fifteen years, but on his son's thirteenth birthday, he had his first flashback. In the weeks that followed, he started having more intense flashbacks and intensive memories about the Vietnam War. He started drinking to "control anxiety."

Bill and his wife were seen in marital therapy starting in 1983. During marital treatment, Bill remembered that he had killed a young Viet Cong soldier who was "about the same age as my son." Bill realized that his son's thirteenth birthday broke his repression about this terrible event. Bill and his wife used marital therapy to find a way to live with their knowledge of this awful event. Bill and Sally learned to be "better parents" and began to volunteer at a youth advocacy agency as a way of giving to the world in "honor" of the young Viet Cong soldier. Bill and Sally eventually adopted two Cambodian refugee children. Sally and Bill are both proud of how they have "honored" Bill's terrible memory and turned it into meaningful "soldier's pay."

Honoring the trauma has been described by Viktor Frankl (1959) as a way to fill the existential-meaning vacuum that often occurs reactive to the trauma experience. Gabriel Marcel (1951) reports that in his opinion, only the manifestation of human love can overcome the negative effects of trauma upon couples and families. To Marcel (1956), honoring the trauma occurs through the human manifestation of availability in the face of trauma, terror, and trauma pain. In our view, honoring the trauma is both an outgrowth of mastery and a facilitating factor in the development of a trauma couple's sense of mastery and control (Lantz, 1974, 1995, 1996).

ART AS EXPERIENTIAL PARTICIPATION WITH TRAUMA COUPLES

In the previous sections of this article, the authors have presented a trauma couple's treatment framework. There is some degree of danger that such a framework may be misunderstood as a treatment "cookbook" if it is not realized that the elements of treatment (holding, telling, mastering, and honoring) unfold in a process of experiential participation (Mullan & Sangiuliano, 1964) between the therapist and the traumatized couple. In our approach to working with traumatized couples, experiential participation is the factor that ensures that treatment remains a process of art.

Traumatized couples frequently come into treatment with fairly rigid ideas and beliefs about how treatment should be "conducted." Often such beliefs inhibit the very change the couple hopes to achieve. The constrictions that the couple attempts to place on the treatment situation often serve as a metaphor for the constrictions that the members of the traumatized couple place upon each other and upon themselves (Lantz, 1996). In this sense, the therapist's insistence upon experiential participation to struggle against the traumatized couple's attempt at constriction models the freedom and flexibility that are required when learning to hold, tell, master, and honor the traumas that have affected their lives (Lantz, 1974, 1993, 1996). The following two clinical illustrations are presented to give a taste of how experiential participation may be used to help a traumatized couple to hold, tell, master, and honor their trauma experiences. The first clinical illustration, a first-person narrative, describes work performed by Dr. Stuck with a traumatized couple who were attempting to learn to love each other and to care for two traumatized children. The second illustration, a partial transcript of a conjoint treatment session, presents work performed by Dr. Lantz with a Vietnam veteran couple. We hope that both clinical examples will show the art of experiential participation as well as the healing elements of holding, telling, mastering, and honoring the trauma experience.

CAROL AND MIKE

I have this couple. An Appalachian couple from the hills of Southeastern Ohio. They are raising two kids. There are Mike, Max, Carol and Sam. Mike is the live-in boyfriend. Max is the suicidal-homicidal seventeen-year-old son. Sam is the fourteen-year-old son who wants to know nothing of his past. Carol is the mother of these two boys. Carol and Mike bring Max to the emergency center. In they come. Max cannot speak. Mom tells me he will speak if she and Mike leave. They leave. Max tells me he wants to have someone killed. I tell him I am sorry he is so hurt and full of pain. Things must be horrible. I notice his hands. I see he has smashed things with his fists. He has scars on his hand. I tell what I see. I ask him of his intent to hit and smash now. He nods. I hand him a teddy bear, and I tell him that I would really-really-really appreciate it if he would not hit me but instead would hit or choke the bear. Would that be suitable for this time? He nods. He tells me of a girl. He wants to kill her stepfather. Max thinks "Paps" is raping this fifteen-year-old girl whom Max says he loves. Max tells me he wants to line up a "Southern Ohio Death." He knows how easily one can have another killed in certain "hollows" that he knows. I believe him. He merely has to make the deal. When he finds out that he is right "for sure" about "Paps," he will have "Paps" killed and then he will kill himself.

I ask Max what has happened to him that causes him to connect so deeply to his girlfriend's pain. He chokes and hits the bear and tells me his tale of blood and abuse. While I listen to him and his story, I want to puke. He tells me what his "father" often did to him.

I wonder what his mom knows. Max tells me that he is afraid to tell her about "Paps." Max is related to "Paps." Paps would kill Max if Max ever "told." Max reports that he trusts Mike, but is afraid that "even Mike" could not help him. We continue (Max and I). Max needs me to understand some more. Max tells me he picks fights and gets beaten nearly to death and does not remember much about the fights other than starting them. He tells me that he cannot stand it if his teachers touch him or tell him what to do. He thinks he needs to die. I ask him if he "disappears" when in these fights or when he is touched. I ask him if he "blacks out." The answer is yes. I am working with a seventeen-year-old who "dissociates" through the use of rage. I talk about how rape victims sometimes leave their bodies. I think he might be leaving his. He slumps down. He nods. I ask him to tell me more. He tells me that I "get it," that "No one has!" I have heard him. I get it. He has started to tell.

Max decides that Carol and Mike should come in. He wants me to help them help him. He wants to tell the story to them. Max wants me to start the story. He will take over as he can. I will help him when he tells me he cannot go on. We will be like tag team wrestlers on Saturday afternoon. We will share his story. Actually, I soon fade out of the story as Max tells it all.

Later I talk to this family about being a 55 gallon drum full to the brim with muck and pain. The drum must be slowly emptied or there will be no room for goodness. Mike looks terrified. I ask him how he is doing, and he tells me he is numb. He understands what Max is saying. I ask how this can be. He tells me what "Paps" once did to him when he was young. He tells me he cannot go on. I look at Carol. She cannot stop her tears. Yet strangely, they are safe for now. Max tells me he will stay alive and will not "make the deal." I ask him to keep the bear.

Carol and Mike call me the next day. They wish to come in as a "couple." We meet. They want to talk. Carol tells me about her memories and dreams. She was brutalized by Max's dad. She was raped. She has been thrown through windows and even driven over by this man in his truck. She has "licked his penis" to stop her children's heads from being smashed on rocks. Again, I want to puke. Carol tells me of passing out from these memories and about vomiting in her abuse-induced coma. I told her the best I can with words. I explain PTSD. I explain (and believe in) the normalcy of her symptoms because of what has happened to her. I explain how she is like her son. Mike and Carol are both in tears. So am I. The family returns in three days, and we continue to talk. Sam starts coming, too.

These are courageous people. Carol tells me she gasps for air. She has something else to tell but she cannot. I ask her about this fear. She is afraid that if she tells, she will lose her mate. She is afraid that Mike will run away. I ask if she can ask Mike if he is going to leave her. Bless this man's pain-filled connection to this woman. He says he doesn't know, but he will try to stay no matter what. He tells her that he loves her. Carol tells Mike that when "we make love," she sees all the men who have raped her. She sees her ex-husband (Max's dad), and she also sometimes sees "Paps" (he has raped her, too). Mike tells Carol that he will hold her until she is drained of pain and that he will not run away. Again, he tells her that he loves her. I am drained and honored and forever and permanently changed because of this courageous couple and their courageous kids. They came to work, and they came to heal.

FRED AND JENNY

Fred and Jenny requested marital therapy after their youngest son left the family to join the Navy. Jenny reported that "we must start fixing the marriage" because she felt that with her son gone, there was no longer any reason to "stay together for the kids." Jenny wanted to "fix" the marriage and would not tolerate its "staying the same." Fred wanted help because "our marriage stinks."

The following transcript segments are from a conjoint therapy session with Fred and Jenny that the couple believes was a turning point in their marriage and their lives. Space constraints prevent sharing the total transcript of the interview, but it is hoped that what is shown will demonstrate the art created during the interview.

W: (To husband) I am a cold fish! No–I'm not. I'm an angry fish! But it's not all my fault. I get so fucking lonely and mad at you sometimes I say fuck it and just go off on my own and other times I just hate you. You are so God damn cold and you were not like that when we were young.
(Therapist's note: This couple dated when they were in high school–before Fred went to Vietnam.)

(long silence)

W: (To husband) Damn . . . it's always been the fucking God damn Vietnam War. It screwed you up!! You were not a cold fish before that fucking war. We have never talked about the war.

H: (with anger–to wife) I did not come here with you to talk about the
    Vietnam War. I came here to talk about our marriage!!!
(Therapist's note: After their exchange, considerable discussion and conflict occurred about the issue of whether or not Vietnam was impacting
upon the relationship and whether Fred would let the therapist help "bring
out" any Vietnam memories that might be "fucking up" the marital relationship. Fred eventually gave the therapist permission to do some memory
work with him and his wife during the conjoint treatment session.)

T: (To husband) Would you be willing to try an experiment? Like a
    gimmick that might bring back something. Something that symbolizes
    things. Maybe it would help, maybe not. How about it? You do this
    experiment with me?

H: (To therapist) What kind of an experiment? Like what?

T: (To husband) We'll just turn around a bit. Face your wife more. Get
    her to face you too . . . then . . . that's good . . . now hold her hands and
    just look at her eyes. Don't do nothing else, just hold her hands and
    look into her eyes. Just do this for a while.

(Long silence as husband and wife look into each others' eyes–this goes
    on about 5 minutes.)

T: (To husband) Okay, good–keep looking at her eyes and holding her
    hands . . . okay, now I want you to keep holding her hand and now
    close your eyes. Close your eyes and keep trying to see your wife's
    face even with your eyes closed.

H: (nods his head)

T: (To husband) Good, just keep your eyes closed and keep the image of
    your wife's face in your mind. Just keep doing this for a while.

(Long silence as husband follows these instructions.)

H: (To therapist) This is nice, but it's getting harder and harder to keep
    my mind on my wife's face; it's like another image wants to come in
    (voice is shaky).

T: (To husband) Okay . . . just keep concentrating on your wife's face for
    a little bit longer.

(silence)

T: (To husband) Okay, now I want you to let go of your wife's image and just let the other image come in. I'm going to count to five, and then just let this other image come over you. 1 . . . 2 . . . 3 . . . 4 . . . okay, 5. Let the new image come in.

H: (Begins sobbing, drops his wife's hand and puts his head in his hands.) Oh, God, it's Bobbie . . . oh, fuck. I don't want to remember this. Oh, God, help me . . . oh, God, I remembered Bobbie but I forgot how awful it was . . . oh, God, forgive me.

H: (Long period of sobbing and rocking.)

W: (Is also sobbing with her husband and is now kissing his left hand.)

T: (To husband) So tell me and your wife about Bobbie. Start putting it into words. Let's open your eyes and take some real long-slow-deep breaths. Look at me or your wife. Take some more long, slow, deep breaths and let's talk about Bobbie. Who was Bobbie?

H: (To therapist and his wife; crying, yet now able to talk) Bobbie was my best friend. I met him when I went to Vietnam. He was in my platoon. We got tight. We were fucking new guys together, and we both made it a long time, but he got zapped. He stepped on a mine, and it just melted him, for Christ sakes. He had parts blown all over the fucking jungle. His body parts dropped on me . . . oh, God . . . from the trees. One minute he's here and the next minute he's slime and parts in the fucking trees dripping all over me . . . oh, God . . . I forgot. (Long period of sobbing and rocking–wife continues to kiss his left hand.)

T: (To husband) Your best friend killed–melted–dripping from trees. God, that is horrible. I'm so sorry. God, I'm sorry. (Therapist starts crying.)

(silence)

H: (To therapist) I really did love him. He was the best friend I ever had. We were tight–God, it hurts.

(Husband again starts sobbing.)

T: (To husband) So tell me and your wife more about Bobbie. Open your eyes and tell your wife about him. Take some deep breaths, real slow–deep. Look at your wife.

(Long silence)

H: (To wife) He was just this great friend. He was nuts. He made me laugh. He had guts. You could count on him to back you up. He did not bug out. He was a friend.

T: (To husband and wife) I seem to remember that your youngest kid . . . the boy . . . is named Robert. Any connection?

H: (To therapist) Yeah . . . he's named after Bobbie. Bobbie was just a fine friend. (Husband puts his head in his hands again and again starts sobbing.)

(Long silence . . . wife comforts and holds her husband.)

T: (To husband) So what happened? Did they just pick him up by copter? Did you body bag him? Did he get a funeral? Where is he now?

H: (still crying) Well, we bagged him. You know, the parts we could find. We did find his tags. We bagged him and then we carried him for miles till we could get a chopper in to take him out. He flew out to graves and registration; that's it. (Again starts deep sobbing.)

T: (To wife) You can start asking some questions when you're ready.

W: (To husband) Baby, I'm so sorry. God, it is awful. I had no idea . . . I'm so sorry. (Wife is crying.)

T: (To husband) You notice she has not bugged out. Did you notice, she didn't run. She just held you and kissed your hand, and she did not run away.

(long silence)

T: (To husband) And she listened to it. She heard it all. Look at her. Look at her eyes. You can tell she heard it all, and it kicked her in the ass, but she did not run away. Look at her.

H: (Looks up at his wife's face and again starts crying.)

(Long silence–husband crying and looking at his wife.)

H: (To therapist) You're right. She didn't back off. It means a lot.

(silence)

H: (To wife) Thank you. Thank you for listening now and for putting up with me all these years . . . Thank you!

(Husband puts his arm around wife and hugs her.) (Wife starts crying.)

(The husband and wife hold each other, cry and whisper to each other for a long period of time–about 10 minutes. During this time, the therapist keeps his mouth shut and does not interrupt or interfere with this important moment of intimacy, otherness, and love that is occurring between husband and wife.)

H: (To therapist) God–thank you. I never felt anything like this in my life. I feel like I've lost 100 pounds off my back. How the hell did you do this . . . how did you know?

T: (To husband) I'm not really sure. It was a hunch. It seemed to fit, so I asked you to do it. And I trusted you and your wife. You're *both* tough!

(silence)

W: (To therapist) Thank you so much. I feel married again.

H: God, that was powerful.

(long silence)

CONCLUSION

In this article the authors have described and illustrated their approach to the art of working with traumatized couples. Such art includes experiential participation between couple and therapist as well as helping the traumatized couple to hold, tell, master and honor their trauma experiences.

REFERENCES

Andrews, E. (1972). Conjoint psychotherapy with couples and families. *Cincinnati Journal of Medicine 53*, 318-319.

Figley, C. (1989). *Helping traumatized families*. San Francisco: Jossey Bass.

Frankl, V. (1969). *From death camp to existentialism*. Boston: Beacon Hill Press.

Lantz, J. (1974). Existential treatment with the Vietnam veteran family. In *Ohio Department of Mental Health Yearly Report* (33-36). Columbus: Ohio Department of Mental Health.

Lantz, J. (1993). *Existential family therapy: Using the concepts of Viktor Frankl.* Northvale: Jason Aronson, Inc.

Lantz, J. (1994A). Mystery in family therapy. *Contemporary Family Therapy 16,* 53-66.

Lantz, J. (1994B). Primary and secondary reflection in existential psychotherapy with couples and families. *Contemporary Family Therapy 16,* 315-327.

Lantz, J. (1994C). Marcel's availability in existential psychotherapy with couples and families. *Contemporary Family Therapy 16,* 489-501.

Lantz, J. (1995). Frankl's concept of time: Existential psychotherapy with couples and families. *Journal Contemporary Psychotherapy 25,* 135-144.

Lantz, J. (1996). Basic concepts in existential psychotherapy with couples and families. *Contemporary Family Therapy 18,* 535-548.

Lindy, J. (1988). *Vietnam: A casebook.* New York: Brunner/Mazel.

Marcel, G. (1951). *Homo viator.* Chicago: Henry Regnery Press.

Marcel, G. (1956). *The philosophy of existence.* New York: The Citadel Press.

Marcel, G. (1963). *The existential background of human dignity.* Cambridge: Harvard University Press.

Mullan, H., and Sangiuliano, I. (1964). *The therapist's contribution to the treatment process.* Springfield: Charles C. Thomas.

Ochberg, F., and Fojtik, K. (1984). A comprehensive mental health service program for victims: Clinical issues and therapeutic strategies. *American Journal of Social Psychiatry 4,* 12-23.

Van Kaam, A. (1959). Phenomenal analysis exemplified by a study of the experience of really feeling understood. *Journal Individual Psychology 15,* 66-72.

Winnicott, D. (1989). Hate in the countertransference. *Voices 25,* 24-34.

Couples and Catastrophe:
Dealing with the Death of a Child
Through Intimacy Therapy

Marcia K. Wiinamaki
David L. Ferguson

SUMMARY. This paper offers a model for integrating Intimacy Therapy into couples' therapy approaches with parents who are experiencing marital distress due to the death of a child. This approach is viewed as adding an important but neglected dimension to commonly used approaches in couples' therapy, emotional responding, thus enhancing the likelihood of a positive outcome. Important concepts of Intimacy Therapy are described, steps to an effective treatment approach are outlined and suggestions are offered for both in-session work and couples' homework. *[Article copies available for a fee from The Haworth Document Delivery Service: 1-800-342-9678. E-mail address: getinfo@haworthpressinc.com]*

One of the most devastating experiences a marriage may sustain is the death of a child. In fact, Brown (1989) has described the death of a child as "life's greatest tragedy" (p. 466). Several reasons for the magnitude of this tragedy have been cited, but perhaps, as Sanders (1979-80) has stated, the most apparent one is that the death of a child seems to violate the

Marcia K. Wiinamaki, PsyD, is a Licensed Clinical Psychologist, and David L. Ferguson, DPhil, is a Licensed Professional Counselor, both at Southwestern Medical Clinic, Christian Counseling and Psychological Services, 5675 Fairview Ave., Stevensville, MI 49127-1099.

[Haworth co-indexing entry note]: "Couples and Catastrophe: Dealing with the Death of a Child Through Intimacy Therapy." Wiinamaki, Marcia K., and David L. Ferguson. Co-published simultaneously in *Journal of Couples Therapy* (The Haworth Press, Inc.) Vol. 7, No. 4, 1998, pp. 19-35; and: *Couples, Trauma, and Catastrophes* (ed: Barbara Jo Brothers) The Haworth Press, Inc., 1998, pp. 19-35. Single or multiple copies of this article are available for a fee from The Haworth Document Delivery Service [1-800-342-9678, 9:00 a.m. - 5:00 p.m. (EST). E-mail address: getinfo@haworthpressinc.com].

© 1998 by The Haworth Press, Inc. All rights reserved.

natural order of the universe. Parents are supposed to die prior to their children. When a child's death is experienced at any age of the child, the expected and "normal" course of life has been violated (Hocker, 1988).

In addition to grief and frequent depression which often occurs in parents who have lost a child due to death, the loss of a child has a profound effect on the marriage relationship as well. DeVries, Lana, and Falck (1994), in an article that both reviewed the literature and laid out a conceptual framework for examining what occurs in the marriage of a bereaved couple, propose that there are a series of factors which influence how the couple experiences grief over the course of their lives. One of the significant factors these authors cite is the role that social support systems play in the resolution of the parental grief Because both partners are experiencing their own suffering at an intense level, it is often difficult for the marriage partners to provide comfort and social support to each other, as Gilbert (1989) and Edelstein (1984) have discussed. Consequently, what is often the most significant social support system in place for the couple, each other, is not available. Furthermore, Gilbert (1989) has documented that, after a child's death, the parents' friends may avoid them in order to not cause them further pain by mentioning the child's name, or because being around the parents of the deceased child may remind them that a tragedy of this nature could potentially occur in their own lives. As a result of this pulling away by friends, "social invitations diminish and social and emotional supports are withdrawn at a time when they are needed the most" (DeVries et al., p. 60).

A qualitative research project which examined the effects of a child's death on the marital relationship of the parents was undertaken by Schwab (1992). Because of its relevance to the topic, we will review the findings of this article in greater depth than the previous articles cited. According to Schwab (1992), six themes emerged from interviews with twenty married couples who had sustained the death of a child in the past four years. The first theme was the husbands' concern and frustration concerning their wives' grief. Along with this concern was a sense of helplessness that they were unable to alleviate this grief. Additional stressors some husbands discussed was their frustration at having to pick up the slack of the household when their wives would be incapacitated or preoccupied with their grief. Wives' anger over their husbands' refusal to express their grief was a second major theme found by the researcher: "Many wives expressed their distress, anger, and disappointment about their husbands' unwillingness to share their grief" (Schwab, 1992, p. 146). Also involving communication changes, the third theme reported was a temporary halt in communication. A common phenomenon reported by many of the couples was that for a time shortly after their child's death, both partners shut themselves off into their own worlds and were not emotionally available to their spouses. According to Schwab (1992): "The highly private nature of grief, its intensity, and the desire not to stir up their spouse's emotions resulted in a virtual cutoff of communication . . ." (p. 148). Not surprisingly, the loss of sexual intimacy constituted the fourth theme in the interviews with the bereaved parents. This loss appeared to be particularly devastating to the husbands because the sexual relationship with their wives was regarded as an important source of comfort, whereas to many of the wives, engaging in sexual activity was viewed as abhorrent and wholly inappropriate given their circumstances. This sexual rejection of the husbands then often triggered fears of also losing the wives, seriously compounding the loss already experienced in the death of their child. A final theme noted by Schwab (1992) was a general irritability between the spouses. Many of those persons interviewed noted that their tempers had "short fuses" as well as their spouses, and furthermore, previous issues were often brought to the surface: ". . . couples' anger, resentment, and irritation were expressed about the issues that had existed before their bereavement and the circumstances surrounding the death and bereavement" (p. 150). A later study which focused on the long-term effects of grief on the marriage after the death of an infant further supports these findings (Gottlieb, Lang, and Amsel, 1996).

As previously mentioned, marriage partners tended to withdraw from each other at different points throughout their grieving process, perhaps at times because of their own pain, and at other times their withdrawal seemed to be motivated out of a desire to reduce their spouse's pain: "When they need one another most, they often find themselves unable to come together or withdrawing into their own private worlds of grief" (Schwab, 1992, p. 153). It is at this point that we believe that Intimacy Therapy will facilitate healing of both partners and the marriage relationship as well; thus, following the presentation of the major tenets of Intimacy Therapy and a brief case scenario of a bereaved couple, we will illustrate the use of Intimacy Therapy in a counseling situation with a couple who has experienced the death of a child. The major tenets of Intimacy Therapy will be applied both within the counseling sessions and outside the session in the form of homework assignments which are designed to increase intimacy within the marriage relationship.

MAJOR TENETS OF INTIMACY THERAPY

The following discussion of the major tenets of Intimacy Therapy have been adapted from *The Pursuit of Intimacy* (Ferguson, Ferguson, Thurman and Thurman, 1993). The most foundational tenet of Intimacy Therapy is that humans are composed of three basic dimensions: spirit, soul, and body. Accordingly, these three dimensions result in various human functions, or consciousness. Thus, the body interacts with the world through the five senses and is "world conscious," while the soul functions through thoughts, feelings, and choices and is "self-conscious." Finally, the dimension concerning "God consciousness" is the spirit, and the spirit functions through conscience, intuition, and worship. Intimacy Therapy strives to address each of these dimensions in marriage counseling.

The next major aspect of Intimacy Therapy concerns motivation: why do people do what they do? According to Intimacy Therapy, a person's raison d'etre is to seek intimacy through meaningful relationships such as within marriage, within the family, and with others. In other words, the major motivator for human beings is relationship. Furthermore, fulfillment in life only results from personally intimate relationships with others. Due to humans being human, however, intimacy with each other and with ourselves is frequently difficult and full of obstacles. Thus, some persons (particularly those who have been deeply wounded through severe abuse and/or neglect) avoid closeness and establish defenses which make it difficult for intimate relationships to occur.

A major purpose for these intimate relationships with meaningful others is meeting the needs we were endowed with; namely, physical, emotional, and spiritual needs. Intimacy needs are best categorized under the heading of emotional needs. Some of the most significant intimacy needs include attention, encouragement, respect, comfort, acceptance, support, security, appreciation, affection, and approval. Intimacy is developed and enhanced through experiencing four major intimacy "ingredients": affectionate caring, vulnerable communication, joint accomplishment, and mutual giving. A crucial element in the first identified ingredient of intimacy, affectionate caring, is the "empathic comforting of identified hurts and needs." Without this empathic comfort, a major hindrance to intimacy will result. Intimacy Therapy seeks to address this issue in the form of "emotional responding," a concept which will be dealt with at greater length in this paper. According to Ferguson, Ferguson, Warren, Warren, and Ferguson (1995):

The family life cycle is considered as bringing predictable challenges to relational intimacy, and thus the need to repeat the "spiral" of intimacy ingredients, beginning with affectionate caring. Thus, the marital stage of mutual giving is challenged by the addition of children to return to affectionate caring, followed by vulnerable communication, joint accomplishment, and again, mutual giving. (p. 358)

Intimacy Therapy holds that one source of problems in living (which may occur in each of the three dimensions–body, soul, and spirit), including marriage and family conflict, are the result of unmet intimacy needs. These unmet needs for intimacy have occurred due to life in a world that is not perfect and being subject to the consequences of others' choices, as well as the suffering which occurs at times as a result of our own faulty choices. Unhealthy thinking, unhealed emotions, and unproductive behaviors are frequently the result of these unmet, or imperfectly met intimacy needs. Consequently, the pattern of unmet needs, unhealthy thinking, unhealed emotions, and unproductive behaviors serves to hinder intimacy and is thus the focus of therapeutic intervention.

Finally, Intimacy Therapy strives to address all origins of hindrances to intimacy, which include the personal, the relational, and the intergenerational. An example of a common intergenerational issue present in many troubled marriages concerns the failure to emotionally "leave" one's family of origin prior to entering into the marriage relationship, thereby hindering relational issues involved in "becoming one" in the marriage.

CASE SCENARIO

Don, age 37, and Sally, age 34, contacted a therapist and initiated therapy approximately 18 months after the accidental death of their 6 year-old son who had drowned. The couple had been married for ten years, and they had one other child, a 4-year-old daughter. Their presenting problems were marital conflict and the sense that they had drifted apart since their son's death. Although both spouses were functioning well in their work roles, their family and marriage relationship had suffered a tremendous strain as a result of the loss of their child. Distressing dreams, irritability, decreased sexual intimacy, and difficulty in communicating were reported by both Don and Sally as symptoms of their marital struggles.

STAGES OF COUNSELING

Intimacy Therapy is a staged approach to marriage counseling, and the four stages which follow describe how marriage counseling is generally conducted in Intimacy Therapy with particular emphasis on Don and

Sally's situation in working through the issues surrounding the death of their son. The basic outline followed by the therapist involves (1) focusing on the couple's grief and assisting them in working through the pain of their loss; (2) focusing on the marital relationship and healing whatever unhealed pain is currently between the two spouses; and (3) focusing on each spouse's relationship with his/her family of origin and working through unhealed hurt that may be in these relationships.

Stage 1

As in object relations therapy as well as Intimacy Therapy, the therapy relationship is a primary tool of the Intimacy Therapist. Because of this emphasis, particular attention is paid to the development of rapport through the offering of empathy and the development of tryst throughout the entire counseling relationship. As Cloud has stated in *Changes That Heal* (1992), most people have been hurt in the context of a relationship, and they need to experience healing in the context of a relationship as well. Intimacy Therapy holds that we are designed to be involved in intimate relationships; therefore, the therapeutic relationship will embody key elements of healthy relationships: empathy, caring, confrontation, honesty, boundaries, vulnerable communication, and attention. In addition to drawing from object relations concepts, the approach of Intimacy Therapy in terms of the therapeutic relationship would look quite similar to that of an existential therapist or interpersonal therapist–the therapist presents him or herself as a fellow traveler on life's journey. The result of this type of therapeutic arrangement is a more egalitarian therapist-client relationship than is generally the case in traditional psychotherapy. Another significant aspect of the therapeutic relationship is the modeling of appropriate intimacy principles and behaviors. Social learning theorists such as Bandura (1969) have demonstrated that observation of a model is a potent method of learning. Thus, the therapeutic relationship will therefore embody the very qualities and principles desired to be cultivated in the client couple.

In addition to setting the tone of the therapeutic relationship discussed above, Stage 1 also focuses on the initial assessment of the individual, the marriage relationship, and intergenerational dynamics. This assessment is accomplished primarily through the interview process. A copy of questions typically used in the initial interview is included at the end of this article. Occasionally, the interview process is supplemented through information obtained from the couple through the use of the "Marital Intimacy Inventory" and "Childhood Questionnaire." The Intimacy Therapist then moves into Stage 2 and chooses interventions appropriate to the information gleaned from the assessment phase of Stage 1.

With Don and Sally, the therapist who is employing Intimacy Therapy would be very active in setting the tone of the therapeutic relationship to be one of empathy. He or she would express appropriately the feelings evoked when hearing the couple's story and the tragedy they have experienced, rather than maintaining a traditional neutral type of stance. In this way, concepts such as "emotional responding" which will be introduced to the couple in a future session will have been modeled for them throughout the entire counseling experience. Furthermore, the therapist's willingness to be transparent with the couple will enhance their development of trust and the therapeutic alliance.

Stage 2

The next aspect of Intimacy Therapy consists of increasing the stability of the marriage relationship. The major intervention at this stage involves an analysis component and an educational component which is tailored to the particular couple's situation. This analysis connects their respective growing up experiences with their marital experiences, particularly the extent to which their intimacy needs have been met or unmet within *their* relationship, to the feelings, thoughts, and behaviors which now occur, particularly in the context of their marriage relationship. Some time may be spent on the "childhood" contributors to current relational issues, but at this stage the greater the severity of the crisis the couple is experiencing, the less time is spent on surfacing childhood pain which may be impacting the marriage relationship and more on identifying how each spouse has contributed to current marital difficulties. This educational component utilizes the metaphor of an "emotional cup," the point being that the accumulation of hurt and pain from relationships produces symptoms such as depression, addictions, anxiety, codependence, rage, and other dysfunctional attempts at coping. While a portion of the accumulated hurt, anger, and pain likely stems from childhood, much more emphasis is placed here on the hurt, anger, and pain stemming from the marriage relationship, or in Don and Sally's case, the pain from the loss of their son which has adversely impacted their marriage relationship. Three emphases comprise this educational component, as needed, depending on the extent to which the couple has had previous exposure to Intimacy Therapy concepts. These three emphases are: (1) determining which intimacy needs are present and which are most important to each partner; (2) what occurs when needs go unmet (symptoms of a "full emotional cup"); and (3) how to empty the "emotional cup" and heal emotional pain through confession, forgiveness, mourning, grieving and receiving comfort.

As Hendrix (1988) and Napier (1988) have argued, the dynamics present in marriage frequently recreate at some level dynamics present in each spouse's family of origin. Because of these dynamics each partner has, in all likelihood, been responsible for wounding his or her partner in ways which he or she has been hurt in the past, compounding the already wounded partner. Therefore, Stage 2 in Intimacy Therapy focuses on increasing the "stability of the marriage relationship as a basis for improved functioning and additional therapeutic intervention" (Ferguson, 1994, p. 264). This stage involves a process of confession and forgiveness for each of the spouses. A detailed educational component is introduced at this stage which outlines the ingredients of confession and forgiveness, respectively, and the couple is given a two-stage homework assignment to accomplish the above.

The therapist utilizing Intimacy Therapy recognizes that healing and growth are processes, not instantaneous events. In order to assist the working through of conflict and the healing of hurt and pain from the past and present, most couples are given homework assignments in the form of handouts. Many of these homework assignments are also available in *Intimate Encounters*, a workbook designed by the founder of Intimacy Therapy, Dr. David Ferguson (1994). The exercises included in the homework, as well as in this workbook, are to be completed separately by each spouse, then a time of focused discussion concerning the exercise is to occur.

Because of the emphasis on communication throughout Intimacy Therapy, the couple is strongly urged to commit to a regular meeting to communicate specifically about the marriage relationship in the form of Marriage Staff Meetings. This format allows the couple a guaranteed time during which they complete the "couple" dimensions of the homework—practicing their communication skills, expressing needs, goals, wants, and desires to their partner in a non-demanding fashion, as well as meeting each spouse's need for focused attention and time that many couples' busy lives make difficult to accomplish on a regular basis, or which they may have been avoiding because of not knowing what to do or how to do it.

Because of Don and Sally's specific type of pain and loss, attention would primarily be focused on their individual grief reactions and eventually move to discussing how their grief has negatively impacted their marriage relationship. Educational interventions with this couple would deal with what is within the realm of normal responses for couples working through the death of their child. As mentioned earlier in this paper, couples who are going through grief over the death of their child frequently withdraw into their own world and are not emotionally available to the other partner. Consequently, a major focus of this phase of therapy would be the identification of each spouse's specific needs, the ways in which these needs are best met, and some training on how to express these needs in a non-demanding manner. According to Guttman (1991):

> In many cases, either the partners are not given to sufficient introspection or the marital relationship has so deteriorated that mutual empathy is very difficult to attain without more dramatic methods. In such instances, the mourning process may be aided by such techniques as: (a) the "empty chair" dialogue with the deceased person; (b) writing a letter to the deceased [a therapeutic letter]; (c) visiting the graveyard in order to say good-bye to [the deceased]; or (d) using a videotape which heightens the awareness of unconscious, repressed anger, sadness, or longing (Paul & Paul, 1982). These interventions may release the mourning process, which can then continue on its own. (p. 86)

Emotional Responding

Along with the identification and expression of needs, particularly intimacy needs, the therapist would also focus on empathy, or "emotional responding." Briefly defined, emotional responding is simply responding to an emotion of another person with an emotion of one's own. For example, if Don notices that Sally looks particularly sad one evening, he might respond to her with the following: "Honey, I notice that you look really sad tonight. I'm hurting for you because I care about you." Because we believe that emotional responding is essential in working through the grieving process, we will now discuss the concept at length as it applies to our couple, Don and Sally.

Although the brief definition of emotional responding appears to be quite simple, the application of it is frequently more complex. The three major components of emotional responding with Don and Sally involve (1) mourning–the expression of sadness concerning a loss; (2) receiving–accepting comfort offered by someone; and (3) giving–providing comfort to another person (see Figure 1). Because Don and Sally may be experiencing their own grief separately at this stage of therapy, it is vital to begin the cycle of mourning, receiving, and giving between the two spouses in order to increase their intimacy and facilitate healing in their own marital relationship as well as their own individual pain and loss suffered. Depending on the characteristics of the bereaved couple, the therapist would direct one of the spouses to begin the cycle by offering comfort to the other spouse. Frequently the wife would be chosen to begin offering comfort, due to many wives' readiness to express their own grief and their

FIGURE 1. Developing Intimacy Skills . . . Emotional Responding

Unproductive Responses

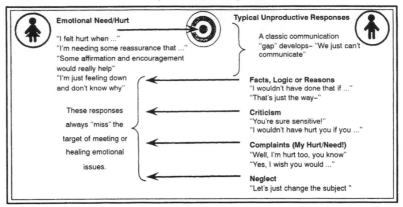

Emotional Responding

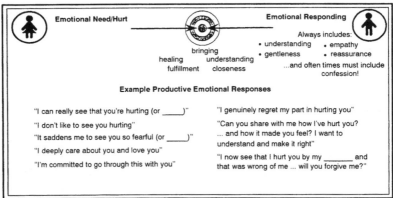

often more keenly developed skills of empathy. However, there are likely many exceptions to this, and the therapist is free to begin with the spouse he or she believes will be most able to express comfort for the mourning of the other spouse.

Forgiveness work may be particularly appropriate for Don and Sally as well. Depending upon the specific set of circumstances surrounding their son's death in a drowning accident, there may be a great deal of guilt and blame that has remained unspoken between the couple. This blame may be directed inward at each spouse, as well as toward the other spouse, for not preventing the accident or placing the child in the situation in the first place. Exercises targeted at expressing one's guilt, as well as fostering openness of feelings between the couple will facilitate intimacy as well as allow the couple to proceed through their own grief processes. As Schwab (1992) has discussed, husbands often feel a sense of inadequacy in dealing with their wives' grief, while the wives are often frustrated by a lack of expression of grief from their husbands. Emotional responding addresses both of these issues which block the marriage partners from completely mourning, receiving comfort, and giving comfort and thus resolving the pain they are experiencing separately and between them as a couple as well

If after sufficient instruction and modeling of the emotional responding process and its components, mourning, receiving, and giving, the couple appears to be stuck, it is important for the Intimacy Therapy clinician to then track down where the hindrances or blockages have occurred. Perhaps because both partners are immersed in their own grieving, there is no giving or receiving of comfort. Many people simply lack the basic relational skills and experience of comforting one another. Thus, focused attention on demonstrating for and equipping the marriage partners in these specific skills using some hypothetical scenarios or vignettes provided by the therapist may be useful. The opportunity to learn to give and receive comfort with other unrelated and less emotionally-charged topics may facilitate the overall grief process.

Unhealed marital hurt is a potential hindrance to the grieving and comforting process. For instance, Sally may be angry with her husband, Don, for being somewhat uninvolved with her and their children and who prioritized work. Consequently, she may experience difficulty in separating her anger toward Don concerning his not spending enough time with their son with her own anger and pain over her own loss of Don's time and attention due to his investment in his work. Because of Sally's anger toward Don that has not been dealt with, her grieving with him may be hindered because of her perception and experience that the marital relationship is not safe. Sally may be quite reluctant to receive comfort from Don if this is the case, because she may not view his comfort as genuine–how could he really care about her when he's been so uninvolved and absent from the family? Here the therapist's role is one of assisting the couple in expressing any unhealed marital hurt that appears to be blocking the mourning/receiving/giving process. Again, Schwab (1992) has indicated that it is quite common for bereaved couples to exhume old issues that seemed to have been settled previous to the death of their child.

Stage 3

Consistent with an object relations framework, Intimacy Therapy holds that the quality of early childhood relationships as well as the meeting of physical and emotional needs are critical for the development of a mature human who may then participate in mutually loving and giving relationships, the most significant of which is the marriage relationship. Thus, Stage 3 of Intimacy Therapy, following the therapist-client relationship, initial assessment, and increased stability phases of marriage counseling, is to facilitate both spouses to reflect first on their families of origin and to determine which needs were met, as well as areas of neglect and/or abuse that may have been present.

During this phase of assessment, the genogram is often employed to clarify the significant issues present in the marriage, as well as family of origin issues which may be contributing significantly to the marriage problems. Of particular interest in this Stage 3, according to Ferguson (1994) are "the Leave-Cleave issues of intergenerational significance which contribute to personal problems in living and marital discord" (p. 264). Throughout his years of experience, Dr. Ferguson has identified that a failure to resolve separation-individuation issues with one's family of origin to a necessary degree prior to marriage is implicated in an overwhelming number of cases of marital conflict and divorce.

Again, due to the nature of Don and Sally's presenting problem, the grief resulting from their son's death and the detrimental impact that has had on their marital relationship, the therapist using Intimacy Therapy principles in this stage of therapy would likely focus on each partner's family of origin, paying particular attention to any unresolved grief and loss issues. The entire grieving and comforting process may be significantly hindered by unhealed childhood and/or other life pain. For example, Don's mourning may have been hindered because of his own view of pain and its expressions as inappropriate or weak which is incongruent with his role as a man. In addition, Don's giving of comfort may be hindered by his own pain from his background of experiencing criticism or neglect when he was hurt. Don's receiving of comfort may be blocked by shame issues provoked by neglect, abuse, or performance-based love that has resulted in his questioning of his own worthwhileness as a person and, by extension, his worthiness of receiving comfort. Potential interventions for both Don and Sally in this phase may be the writing of therapeutic letters to family members with whom there is a loss or has been a death. The couple may even be encouraged to write their own letters to their son and read them in the session. The therapist will facilitate the spouses to provide comfort to each other, as well as encourage the development and use of their other social support networks, including family members, friends, co-workers, and perhaps joining a support group for parents who have lost children to death.

As discussed in the early portion of this paper, couples such as Don and Sally frequently experience an increased level of irritability with each other as they progress through the grief process. In addition, it is likely that issues previous to the death of their child which had not been completely worked through may emerge at a later time. Because the couple may not be communicating as well as they had prior to the death of their child, these issues may appear to be more difficult and the couple may experience a significant amount of frustration and hopelessness as these issues surface. Consequently, the therapist should be alert for struggles in their communication and be prepared to teach interventions which focus on healthy communication, even if the couple once possessed excellent communication skills.

Stage 4

The final phase of marriage counseling in Intimacy Therapy involves the implementation of the "Becoming One Disciplines." These disciplines "help ensure relational intimacy, personal maturity, and positive mental health" (Ferguson, 1994, p. 265). Included in this Stage are such joint projects as establishing a vision for your marriage (and family, if applicable) through setting goals which encompass the following areas of life: spiritual, marriage, family, household, financial, career/domestic, and personal/social. Couples in this stage are encouraged to develop goals while getting away together on a goal-setting retreat with a specific agenda.

Following the goal-setting phase of Stage 4, couples are encouraged to relate intimately with each other on each of three levels; namely, in body, soul, and spirit. Consequently, marriage partners, in order to be fully intimate with each other, must develop the friendship aspect of their relationship (soul), the sexual aspect of their relationship (body), and the spiritual aspect of their relationship (spirit).

According to Intimacy Therapy, the friendship aspect of the marriage relationship consists primarily of making time for each other through dating, the development of common interests, the initiation of appreciation, affection, and interest in one's spouse, and warm, eager greetings upon seeing each other. As mentioned previously, marriage staff meetings are crucial in creating time spent together. The marriage staff meeting is a two-hour priority meeting each week during which such aspects of marriage as calendar coordination, family goals, parenting plans (if children are a part of the family), listening times for one or both, productive criticism and hopes for the future, as well as the opportunity to express appreciation for who one's spouse is and for what he or she has done.

Promoting sexual intimacy is the focus of relating to one's spouse at the physical level. Rather than viewing sex as something couples "do" or "have," Intimacy Therapy holds that the sexual relationship is primarily sharing one another's presence in being together and becoming sexually one. An important tool in Intimacy Therapy used to increase sexual intimacy is the "Love Map." The Love Map is an exercise which first focuses attention on the four major hindrances to sexual intimacy, then provides each spouse the opportunity to express his/her ideal sexually intimate times with his/her spouse on paper. Following this portion of the exercise, the spouses get together to share vulnerably with each other the desires expressed on their Love Maps. At the conclusion of this time of deep and caring sharing, the spouses are to then schedule two times of intimacy set aside to fulfill both spouses' Love Maps.

The third level of relating intimately with one's spouse involves the development of closeness in the spiritual arena, both at the individual and marriage relationship levels. To begin the process of spiritual closeness in the marriage relationship, it is suggested that the couple choose a goal which encourages their joint spiritual development. Such goals may involve church attendance together, regular Scripture reading, or the establishment of a daily meditational time. An exercise designed to facilitate a spiritual focus for the couple is the "Journal of Gratefulness" which is basically a diary which chronicles the date, the family member involved, the means of blessing, and how the appreciation for the blessing was expressed. Finally, the couple is encouraged to develop intimacy with others, particularly through meaningful service and involvement together in relationships in the local church and in the community.

In this phase of therapy, it will be important to address Don and Sally's relationship with each other, especially the sexual aspect. As previously mentioned, several researchers have identified the bereaved couple's sexual relationship as potentially fragile (Gottlieb, Lang, and Amsel, 1996; and Schwab, 1992). Common gender differences in the grief process should be pointed out by the therapist, which will help normalize the added stress that the loss of a positive sexual relationship between the couple may represent. Further, this discussion may calm the fears of both partners, who may be concerned about the future of the marriage.

The friendship aspect of the marriage relationship also should serve as a focus of therapy in this phase of treatment of Don and Sally. The marriage staff meeting and regularly scheduled dates will allow the couple to spend positive time with each other and will also prevent the surviving child from dominating the attention of both parents to the exclusion of the marital relationship. In addition, the time the couple spends together may serve to re-bond them following the trauma they have experienced which has contributed to them drifting apart.

The spiritual aspect of their marriage is yet another focus of attention in treatment. Because of the existential impact of their son's death on Don and Sally, they will likely be calling into question foundational spiritual and religious beliefs. While the therapist may recommend that the couple speak with a clergy member, it is vital that the therapist be open to allowing the couple to work through these major spiritual issues within the sessions as well. To curtail such discussions will likely seriously undermine the therapeutic alliance and impede the couple's progress in therapy. The spiritual aspect of their relationship may also be attended to by suggesting that the couple become involved, when appropriate, in a joint charity or ministry project. This endeavor will serve to enhance the couple's intimacy, as well as provide them the opportunity to be productive to society in a way that may very well bolster their own self-esteems following the devastating loss they have experienced.

MAJOR FOCI OF INTIMACY THERAPY

By way of review, the major foci of Intimacy Therapy are as follows:

1. An emphasis on a warm, empathic, egalitarian therapist-client relationship, as well as on the assessment of the individuals, the marriage relationship, and intergenerational dynamics through the Marital Intimacy Inventory and Childhood Questionnaire;
2. Psychoeducational components which involve making the connection between unmet marriage needs and current symptom patterns, specifically through the metaphor of the emotional cup, with the concept that if some needs were unmet in childhood, pain in the marriage would be even greater than if those early needs had been appropriately taken care of;
3. Additional education concerning the process of comforting one's spouse for the hurt and pain of the marriage, then putting this new skill into effect;
4. Teaching concerning confession and forgiveness, with each spouse confessing his/her offense to one's spouse, experiencing forgiveness, and then reversing roles and continuing the process;
5. Appropriate attention to unmet childhood emotional needs and how these needs may have impacted their current relationships; and

6. The use of a workbook and exercises which serve to both educate and provide experiential and emotional components which consolidate and maintain the skills and insights gained in therapy. Examples of these skills include the recognition of one's needs, the recognition of one's spouse's needs, how to present needs and desires in a non-demanding, non-critical manner, and how to effectively meet one's spouse's needs.

ADDITIONAL POTENTIAL APPLICATIONS OF INTIMACY THERAPY

Because of the emphasis of Intimacy Therapy on the concept of unmet needs in childhood which result in a variety of maladaptive coping strategies that detrimentally affect interpersonal relationships in general, and the marriage relationship in particular, this type of therapy approach is applicable to a wide variety of presenting problems. Examples of some common marital problems which have been addressed by Intimacy Therapy include the following:

1. infidelity;
2. lack of intimacy;
3. enmeshment with family of origin;
4. poor conflict resolution skills;
5. poor communication skills;
6. domestic violence situations;
7. drug, alcohol, and sexual addictions;
8. sexual problems as a result of incest;
9. codependency.

REFERENCES

Bandura, A., Blancard, E.B., and Ritter, B. (1969). The relative efficacy of desensitization and modeling approaches for inducing behavioral, affective, and attitudinal change. *Journal of Personality and Social Psychology, 13*, 173-199.

Brown, F.H. (1989). The impact of death and serious illness on the family life cycle, in *The Changing Family Life Cycle: A Framework for Family Therapy (2nd Edition)*, Carter, E., and McGoldrick, M., eds., Allen & Bacon, Boston, 457-482.

Cloud, H. (1992). *Changes that heal*. Grand Rapids: Zondervan Publishing House.

DeVries, B., Lana, R.D., and Falck, V.T. (1994). Parental bereavement over the life course: a theoretical intersection and empirical review. *Omega*, 29(1), 47-69.

Edelstein, L. (1984). *Maternal bereavement: coping with the unexpected death of a child*. New York: Praeger.

Ferguson, D.L., Ferguson, T., Thurman, C., and Thurman, H. (1994). *Intimate encounters: A practical guide to discovering the secrets of a really great marriage*. Nashville: Thomas Nelson Publishers.

Ferguson, D., Ferguson, T., Warren, P., Warren, V., and Ferguson, T. (1995). *Parenting with intimacy workbook: A practical guide to building and maintaining great family relationships*. Wheaton, IL: Victor Books.

Gottlieb, L.N., Lang, A., and Amsel, R. (1996). The long-term effects of grief on marital intimacy following an infant's death. *Omega*, 33(1), 1-19.

Guttman, H.A. (1991). Parental death as a precipitant of marital conflict in middle age. *Journal of Marital and Family Therapy*, *17(1)*, 81-87.

Hendrix, H. (1988). *Getting the love you want: A guide for couples*. New York: HarperPerennial.

Hocker, W.V. (1988). Parental loss of an adult child. *Grief and the loss of an adult child*, Margolis, O.S. et al., eds., New York: Praeger, 37-49.

Livneh, H., Antonak, R.F., and Maron, S. (1995). Progeria: medical aspects, psychosocial perspectives, and intervention guidelines. *Death studies, 19*, 433-452.

Napier, A. (1988). *The fragile bond*. New York: HarperPerennial.

Sanders, C. (1979-80). A comparison of adult bereavement in the death of a spouse, child and parent. *Omega*, 10(4), 303-322.

Schwab, R. (1992). Effects of a child's death on the marital relationship: a preliminary study. *Death Studies*, 16, 141-154.

The Impact of Parental Abduction on the Couple

Geoffrey L. Greif

SUMMARY. The abduction of a parent's child by the other parent can be an extremely heart-wrenching experience. Not only are the child's whereabouts and safety placed in doubt, the searching parent's life is thrown into turmoil. This case example describes the impact that the long-term abduction of a mother's son had on the mother's ability to maintain a relationship as a member of a new couple. *[Article copies available for a fee from The Haworth Document Delivery Service: 1-800-342-9678. E-mail address: getinfo@haworthpressinc.com]*

Occasionally, and often in the most acrimonious divorce situations in which custody of children is in dispute, one parent or family member threatens or actually kidnaps a child and goes into hiding. If such a catastrophic event occurs, it throws the family system into enormous turmoil. Not only is there a significant impact on the child's development when he or she is in hiding and out of touch with the usual sources of support, the parent left behind also suffers. This article discusses one such situation: that of a couple in which the mother's son was abducted by her husband from a first marriage and the difficulty the couple had in sustaining their relationship.

Geoffrey L. Greif, DSW, is Associate Dean and Professor for the School of Social Work, University of Maryland, Baltimore, 525 W. Redwood St., Baltimore, MD 21201.

[Haworth co-indexing entry note]: "The Impact of Parental Abduction on the Couple." Greif, Geoffrey L. Co-published simultaneously in *Journal of Couples Therapy* (The Haworth Press, Inc.) Vol. 7, No. 4, 1998, pp. 37-46; and: *Couples, Trauma, and Catastrophes* (ed: Barbara Jo Brothers) The Haworth Press, Inc., 1998, pp. 37-46. Single or multiple copies of this article are available for a fee from The Haworth Document Delivery Service [1-800-342-9678, 9:00 a.m. - 5:00 p.m. (EST). E-mail address: getinfo@haworthpressinc.com].

© 1998 by The Haworth Press, Inc. All rights reserved.

THE CONTEXT OF PARENTAL ABDUCTION

Child custody disputes and marital breakups tear at the core of the family and place children and parents in impossible situations in which there rarely are resolutions satisfactory to everyone. At the extreme are those relationship problems or custody disputes that include a kidnapping and other illegal actions. If parental abduction is defined broadly to include any unauthorized taking or retaining of a child, most incidents are resolved within a few days, usually after either a legal authority or a lawyer has contacted the abducting parent, or after the abducting parent returns the child without legal intervention (Greif & Hegar, 1993). Finkelhor et al. (1990) estimate that 10 percent of abductions last longer than a month. In these longer term situations, the whereabouts of the abductors and children are either unknown or is known only generally by the searching parent. In general, it is rare for children to experience serious harm while in hiding (Finkelhor, Hotaling, & Sedlak, 1991).

Estimates of the number of child snatchings undertaken by family members in the U.S. have reached as high as 350,000 annually (Finkelhor, Hotaling, & Sedlak, 1990), though anecdotal research places the number at lower levels. Family abduction (often referred to as parental abduction as parents are more apt to abduct than other family members, like grandparents or aunts and uncles) comprises by far the largest proportion of the child kidnapping problem, while stranger abduction is estimated to occur less than 5,000 times a year (Finkelhor et al., 1990).

Parental abductions occur within the context of failing or failed adult relationships. A parent snatches a child either as a marital or nonmarital relationship is breaking up, or within a period of time ranging from a few days to a few years afterward. Traumas in general clearly have an impact on a relationship. Recent research shows that spousal support can moderate this impact (Broman, Riba, & Trahan, 1996). Whereas some attention has focused on adults' capacity to build new relationships after divorce, the consequences of this specific related traumatic event on a newly forming couple have been virtually ignored.

In these situations, the toll on the searching parent, the focus of this article, can be enormous. It is rare that a relationship ends without some rancor and hurt. Open wounds are left that are often slow to heal. When an abduction occurs, any attempts at self-healing cease as the abducting parent, representing the failed relationship, becomes a larger than life presence, impossible to forget or ignore. If the abductor is viewed as a "bad" person (not always the case), the situation is exacerbated as the searching parent fears significant harm may befall the missing child. Long-term abductions present the possibility for the most significant disruptions to occur.

More often than not, searching parents perceive that they have been more involved with the upbringing of the child than the abductor when the child is taken. They are usually the parent who has custody after the divorce, though sometimes it is the custodial parent who leaves the area, either fearing that the child will be taken by the other parent or fearing for the child's well-being during visitation with the other parent. Thus, with the loss of the child, they are confronted not only with fears about the child's well-being but the filial deprivation that results from not seeing a loved one that they have had meaningful responsibility for raising.

Studies of Searching Parents

A handful of research has examined the emotional state of the searching parent. One study of 65 such parents found them to be experiencing sleep disorders, anxiety, depression, despair, and feelings of helplessness (Janvier, McCormick, & Donaldson, 1990). Another study of 17 searching parents revealed some levels of pathology but few parents who were suffering it to a severe extent (Forehand, Long, Zogg, & Parrish, 1989).

The largest survey of the population to date was of 371 parents whose children were kidnapped, half of whom had recovered their children by the time of the survey (Greif & Hegar, 1993). Three-quarters of the children were six or younger at the time of the snatching and the average length of time the children were gone was over a year. The most common reactions experienced by these parents were: feelings of loss–85%; feelings of rage–77%; loss of sleep–75%; loneliness–69%; and fearfulness–57%. Slightly over half reported receiving mental health treatment, most commonly for depression (Greif & Hegar, 1991) and a handful were hospitalized for psychiatric treatment (Greif & Hegar, 1993), proving the need for practitioners to be cognizant of the issues these parents face. In addition, and relevant to the case study to follow, over half of the searching mothers (significantly more than the searching fathers) reported being the victims of domestic violence prior to the abduction. Finally, females were more apt than males to believe that the abduction was undertaken to hurt them, that revenge rather than a desire to be with the children was the motivating factor (Hegar & Greif, 1991). Revenge has been cited in other studies also as a motivating factor (Sagatun & Barrett, 1990). This also will be represented in the case example.

What tasks do searching parents face? Perhaps the most difficult is the decision about how strenuously to search for one's child. Naturally, a parent spends every waking hour in pursuit when the child is first missing. But what happens as the days turn to weeks and then to months and the child is still not recovered? The ability to balance the need to search while

maintaining stability in one's personal and work life is often excruciating-
ly difficult. In addition, searching parents have to learn whether to include
or exclude other family members in the search process. Some parents want
their own parents' involvement. Others though, find such help intrusive as
it reenacts for them past conflicts. For example, the parent's parents may
have been initially opposed to the relationship between the parent and the
abductor. An "I told you so" attitude from the parents becomes a reminder
of the searching parent's failure. Left-behind siblings also need an explanation as to what their role can be in the search process. For a child who
was not taken, feelings of rejection, relief, and guilt are common. An
additional burden on the searcher is learning how to work with legal
authorities. The FBI, local police, lawyers, and support networks like the
National Center for Missing and Exploited Children all may be involved in
the search efforts and be placing demands on the parent while attempting
to be helpful. In the end, the searching parent is pulled in many directions
while also trying to keep life as stable as possible.

CASE EXAMPLE

The following couple came to me for consultation following the abduction of the mother's four year-old son by the son's father 18 months prior
to the interview. They were familiar with my colleague's and my work in
the area of parental kidnapping and were also visiting the FBI in Washington, DC to try and coordinate search efforts. The initial interview lasted 90
minutes and was videotaped. It was preceded by a lengthy discussion in a
more informal atmosphere. Following the interview, the couple contacted
us three more times seeking further assistance.

Vera is a 30 year old white woman who was married to Manny for three
years. The couple met while in graduate school. Vera was American born
and is close to her parents. Manny is from a South American country and,
even though he was living in the U.S., maintained strong ties to his native
country, often visiting his relatives there for extended periods of time. The
marriage was stormy from the beginning and produced one child, Dick.
The couple broke up when Dick was one and Vera assumed custody with
Manny having sporadic visitation.

Six months after the breakup, Vera began a serious relationship with
Dave, a white man in his early 30s who worked as a counselor. Dave
moved in with Vera and Dick a few months later and became, to a large
extent, a surrogate father. When Dave moved in, Manny's desire for contact with Manny increased exponentially. He began to drop by unan-
nounced, would take Dick out for longer periods of visitation than were

originally agreed upon, and engaged in angry confrontations with Vera about how Dick was being raised. Vera became afraid of Manny's outbursts and began to fear for her own safety.

Then the ultimate happened. Following one weekend visitation, Manny and Dick did not return. By Monday morning, Vera was calling everyone she could think of in an attempt to locate her son. Finally, she called the police and the FBI and filed a missing person's report. The obvious points of exit were monitored, the airports and train stations, but there were no signs of them. Vera did not believe that Manny cared enough for Dick to want to raise him. Rather she believed he was motivated by a sense of machismo about another man raising his child and that the only way to gain control and a sense of revenge was to kidnap.

While some abductors communicate occasionally with the searching parent to give reassurance that the child is being well taken care of, no such message was sent. Vera heard nothing.

The Toll on Vera and Dave

Over the next months, Vera and Dave spent an enormous amount of time and energy searching for Dick. It is this period that is the most difficult for a couple and their evolving relationship. Who picks up what responsibilities? How will limited resources be spent? As mentioned earlier, how much time should a parent spend searching? How much emotional support is needed? For Vera and Dave, their opinion about Dick's well-being colored their search efforts. My consultation with them focused directly on these issues–they wanted to learn from me how Dick would fare living with his father and whether Dick would still remember them if he was located. These were, of course, two impossible questions to answer given the lack of information we were working with and the developmental changes that Dick was experiencing.

They described Dick as being very loving and as being close to both Vera and Dave. They brought a video tape of happy times the three of them had together. But they also presented a dark side to the scenario. Manny was described as loving but "diabolical." Vera said that he was very smart and would be difficult to locate. Even more darkly she worried that even if she recovered Dick that Manny might come and kill her someday. She felt she was locked into a lifelong struggle with him until Dick was old enough to be independent of both of them. She wondered if she should just give up the search completely, if that would be the only way she would ever achieve peace. While Dave expressed great rage toward Manny for what he had done, Vera felt little anger toward him. Perhaps she needed a way to deny her own role in choosing him as a husband and, by being less angry at him she was giving herself a break.

During the interview, Vera talked eloquently about the strain the abduction had on her relationship with Dave while also referring to him as the man she loved. "I know this is very hard on Dave. Sometimes I get angry at him when I know I am really angry that Dick is missing." "Dave, can you tell the difference between when she is mad at you for what you did and mad at you for something else?" I interjected at this point. "Yes," Dave replied, "but it is very hard." Vera took his hand at this point. "I know Dave is taking care of the home while I am taking care of the search and it is not always fair to him," she responded. She talked further about needing time to search while also reserving time to continue her graduate studies, that her life could not just stop until Dick was located. Her studies provided respite for her, in fact, a chance to try and forget for a few hours that her son was missing. "But he is always in my thoughts," she said.

The discussion returned to how I thought Dick was faring living with Manny and being in hiding. I gave a broad brush stroke of life for children on the run. I said that children who are torn away from the parent they are more emotionally attached to are going to have a harder time than children who are taken by the primary parent. I explained that Manny could make it very easy on Dick by not changing his name and by reassuring him that his mother still loved him even though she was not seeing him at the moment. But Manny could also make life very hard for Dick by telling him that Vera did not love him or had been killed.

The intervention I attempted at this point was one that I find helps parents to deal with imponderables. I ask them, "What fantasy can the two of you construct together as to Dick's well-being that will allow you both to continue to search and to find pleasure in your life while you search?" It had to be a construction that was true to their beliefs and yet would enable them to be able to occasionally go to a movie and enjoy it, a reference to an earlier part of the discussion, without feeling they had to leave and check with yet another missing children's organization. They were told they did not have to agree with the other partner's fantasy. They discussed their initial reactions to the question and, as the session ended, continued to think about the question. They both seemed relieved at the end of the session and vowed to stay in touch.

In fact, Vera wrote me a letter a few weeks later thanking us for the support and saying how much she learned. She was continuing the search and stated, "Sometimes it feels like we're close but things don't look very good right now. We've hired a psychic! Everything she said was brilliantly logical, sensible and helpful, but so far, none of the predictions had come true . . . But Dave and I are managing well despite the circumstances.''

Then, six months later, I received a frantic but joyous call from Vera. Dick had been located in Manny's native South American country with the help of an ad in the newspaper and Vera and Dave had been given permission by the government to visit him. They were flying out the next morning and wanted to know, for the reunion, what they should bring, how they should act, and what they should say about where they had been. They had no idea what Dick had been told. Dave wanted to know if he should be present for the initial visit with Dick.

Two weeks later they called again and said they had visited, that Dick did remember them after some initial confusion, but that they had left without him. The government had not recognized their right to him, a common occurrence if the country has not signed the Hague Convention on the Civil Aspects of International Child Abduction (Girdner & Hoff, 1994). Even their departure was problematic as Manny bribed the airport officials who refused to let them fly out. Fearing for their safety, they rented a car and drove across the border.

A new stage of Vera and Dave's relationship began. Dick was no longer missing; he was now the child they could not bring home. They were elated and saddened at the same time. It was a relief to a large extent but also marked the introduction of a new set of burdens on the other. They were maddeningly close to him while still being a continent away. They had one foot in South America and one foot in the U.S.

Whereas they had constructed a way to stay together for the search, where the common enemy was the abduction and Manny, they now had to change gears and deal with a radical shift in their circumstances. Manny was still in the driver's seat though they had won round two by locating Dick. The new demands the couple was asked to withstand proved too much. They broke up. Dave left but Vera, who told me about the end of the relationship, wondered if she drove him away. Dave continues to be interested in Dick but has no ongoing contact as Dick still lives on a different continent.

Vera's concerns about Dick's well-being have not been quieted by his being located. Shortly after the O.J. Simpson case became public, she called me, extremely concerned that Manny may come and kill her or kill Dick as she believed O.J. had done to his wife. She asked that I call Manny in South America and find out if he intended to do any harm. As I had no relationship with Manny and doubted that I could learn anything even if I had, I refused. That was the last contact I had with her.

DISCUSSION AND CONCLUSION

This couple was living happily and raising Vera's son when he was abducted. By their own accounts, the strain of the abduction caused the end of their relationship. It is easy to state that if the relationship had been strong enough it would have survived. But that ignores the nature of this particular abduction, which pulled at Vera and Dave for well over two years and which forced them to cope with two different variations of the kidnapping: the searching period and the locations-but-inability-to-regain-custody period.

With a couple coping with an abduction, one member is always going to be more angry at the abductor than the other (Dave); one member is going to want to spend more time and money on the search than the other (Vera); one member will be more dedicated to the maintenance of the relationship than the other (Dave), etc. If the couple's relationship becomes vulnerable, unresolved issues directly related to the previous relationship will affect the present. For example, Dave and Vera acknowledge that she is sometimes angry at Dave for issues that are related to Manny. In such a tango, *any* expression of anger can then be denied by Dave. All spontaneity is removed from their interactions as Dave has to process (more than usually occurs) if Vera should be angry at him or if he is just an easy target. If he chooses to dismiss her anger, a circularity begins whereby she becomes angry at him for ignoring her feelings.

By way of a second example of how a previous relationship affects the current one, Vera could interpret Dave's unwillingness to expend every hour in the search as not valuing Dick while he interprets her wishes to search all the time as not valuing him and their relationship. In this context, every mention of Dick could be seen by Dave as a way of minimizing the adults' relationship while Dave may react in a way that makes his behavior seen unresponsive to Vera's needs. Eventually such differences can pull couples apart.

If those differences do not, then a second blow to the relationship, e.g., having to negotiate with Manny and his government around custody and visitation, might. Couples can sometimes deal with one catastrophic event. But when a second one comes, it can push them past the point of coping. The location of Dick certainly removed much of the doubt and pain associated with a missing child. But it opened up new areas of concern, as attested to by Vera's fears of reprisal stirred up by the O.J. Simpson case. Dynamically, one door was closed but another was opened which required a new set of coping responses. The couple was worn out and could no longer muster the response needed to stay together.

I would not have predicted at the first meeting that this couple would break up. I can, with hindsight and their input, say it was the second stressful event that precipitated the split. For other couples, it may actually be the cessation of the initial catastrophic event, particularly if it is on-going as this was, which cause the breakup. Once the couple no longer has an outside crisis to join forces against, they may have no impetus to stay together. The crisis may serve to tamp down bubbling relationship prob-lems. The catastrophe may, in fact, prevent a breakup as long as it is operative.

Could Dave have left Vera before Dick had been recovered? If he had, it would have meant that Manny had defeated their relationship, that he had won in his quest to wreak havoc on their lives. If Dave were "a nice guy," it would also have been difficult to leave Vera when she was still in the crisis situation of searching. Only when Dick was located could Dave perhaps give himself permission to leave. It could be the same for other couples. Only when the abducting parent has been found and is no longer interfering with the relationship as he or she had been, can the couple then honestly deal with each other and stop guarding against the abductor's intrusion.

NOTE

The initial interview with this couple was discussed in Greif (1996). Since that interview, new information is available that pertains to the long-term negative effects of this kind of stress on the couple.

REFERENCES

Broman, C.L., Riba, M.L., & Trahan, M. 1996. Traumatic events and marital well-being. *Journal of Marriage and the Family, 58*, 908-916.

Finkelhor, D., Hotaling, G., & Sedlak, A. 1990. *Missing, abducted, runaway and throwaway children in America: Numbers and characteristics.* Washington, DC: Department of Justice.

Finkelhor, D., Hotaling, G., & Sedlak, A. 1991. Children abducted by family members: A national household survey of incidence and episode characteris-tics. *Journal of Marriage and the Family, 53*, 805-817.

Forehand, R., Long, N., Zogg, C., & Parrish, E. 1989. Child abduction: Parent and child functioning following return. *Clinical Pediatrics, 28*, 311-316.

Girdner, L. & Hoff, P. 1994. *Obstacles to the recovery and return of parentally abducted children.* Washington, DC: Office of Juvenile Justice and Delinquen-cy Prevention.

Greif, G.L. 1996. Coping with the crisis of a parentally abducted child: A crisis intervention and brief treatment perspective. In A. Roberts (Ed.). *Crisis management & brief treatment: Theory, technique, and applications*, pp. 105-122. Chicago: Nelson-Hall.

Greif, G.L. & Hegar, R.L. 1991. Parents whose children are abducted by the other parent: Implications for treatment. *American Journal of Family Therapy, 19,* 215-225.

Greif, G.L. & Hegar, R.L. 1993. *When parents kidnap: The stories behind the headlines.* New York: The Free Press.

Hegar, R.L. & Greif, G.L. 1991. Abduction of children by their parents: A survey of the problem. *Social Work, 36,* 421-426.

Janvier, R.F., McCormick, K., & Donaldson, R. 1990. Parental kidnapping: A survey of left-behind parents. *Juvenile and Family Court Journal,* 41, 1-8.

Sagatun, I. & Barrett, L. 1990. Parental child abduction: The law, family dynamics, and legal system responses. *Journal of Criminal Justice, 18,* 433-442.

Elective Pediatric Amputation: Couples at a Crossroads

Patrick J. Morrissette
Debra Morrissette
Michelle Naden

SUMMARY. Couples who enter into the deliberation process regarding elective amputation of an infant's limb face an enormous challenge and can experience a myriad of emotions. Such emotions can disrupt the couple's typical interactional pattern, strain their relationship and hinder parenting efforts. If preventative or remedial action is not taken to resolve contentious or anxiety producing issues that arise during the decision making process, conflict can emerge and threaten the intimate relationship. The purpose of this article is to briefly describe congenital pseudarthrosis and discuss intrapsychic, interpersonal, and ecological factors that couples typically encounter while grappling with decisions that have major ramifications for their infant. Along with case vignettes, recommendations that are designed to assist couples during the deliberation process are provided. *[Article copies available for a fee from The Haworth Document Delivery Service: 1-800-342-9678. E-mail address: getinfo@haworthpressinc.com]*

When faced with having to make medical decisions for their children, parents can expect to experience a certain level of stress fueled by a sense of uncertainty and trepidation. When having to contend with medical decisions that will have a definite and significant impact on their offspring's life,

Patrick J. Morrissette and Debra Morrissette are affiliated with Montana State University-Billings.
Michelle Naden is affiliated with Seattle Pacific University.

[Haworth co-indexing entry note]: "Elective Pediatric Amputation: Couples at a Crossroads." Morrissette, Patrick J., Debra Morrissette, and Michelle Naden. Co-published simultaneously in *Journal of Couples Therapy* (The Haworth Press, Inc.) Vol. 7, No. 4, 1998, pp. 47-62; and: *Couples, Trauma, and Catastrophes* (ed: Barbara Jo Brothers) The Haworth Press, Inc., 1998, pp. 47-62. Single or multiple copies of this article are available for a fee from The Haworth Document Delivery Service [1-800-342-9678, 9:00 a.m. - 5:00 p.m. (EST). E-mail address: getinfo@haworthpressinc.com].

© 1998 by The Haworth Press, Inc. All rights reserved.

however, the stress experienced by the couple heightens markedly and directly influences their relationship (Albrecht, 1995; Rolland, 1994; Varni & Setoguchi, 1993). This may prove especially true in situations where the prognosis for recovery is tenuous. Early studies pertaining to congenital heart disease (Apley, Barbour, & Westmacom, 1967; Lavigne & Ryan, 1979; Linde, Rasof, & Dunn, 1970) and studies regarding congenital or acquired limb deficiencies (Varni & Setoguchi, 1993) demonstrate how these medical conditions can influence and disrupt marital and family relationships.

This paper provides a preliminary exploration into the lives of couples whose infant had been diagnosed with congenital pseudarthrosis and where elective amputation was considered a viable alternative. While doing so, intrapersonal, interpersonal, and ecological factors impacting the couple relationship were examined and consequential issues were discussed. The case examples involved five rural-based couples who sought outpatient consultation regarding psychosocial issues relating to their circumstances. The mean age of the couples was 33 years. Each couple had been married for approximately six years and other children were present in each family.

CONGENITAL PSEUDARTHROSIS: AN OVERVIEW

Congenital pseudarthrosis of the tibia (CPT) is a rare disorder that has received substantial attention within the medical literature (Andrew, Bassett, & Schink-Ascani, 1991; Anderson, Schoenecker, Sheridan, & Rich, 1992; Crossett, Beaty, Betz, Warner, Clancy & Steel, 1988; Morandi, Zembo, & Ciotti, 1989; Paley, Catagni, Argnani, Prevot, Bell, & Armstrong, 1991; Paterson, 1989; Rajacich, Bell, & Armstrong, 1991; Strong & Wong-Chung, 1991). CPT was described almost 300 years ago and remains one of the least understood and difficult conditions to treat in orthopedic surgery (Crossett, Beaty, Betz, Warner, Clancy, & Steel, 1988; Paterson, 1989). Neurofibromatosis and fibrous dysplasia are known associated conditions; however, the etiology and pathogenesis of CPT are inexact (Paley, Catagni, Argnani, Prevot, Bell, & Armstrong, 1991). According to Anderson (1972) the incidence of CPT is one in 140,000 newborns and includes "all congenital fractures of the tibia as well as pseudarthrosis of the tibia arising after a pathologic fracture in a tibia with congenital anterior angulation" (p. 44). Although surgical intervention designed to preserve the limb has improved over the past 40 years, there remains a high failure rate (Paterson, 1989). Forms of surgical intervention involve: bone grafting, internal and external fixation, electrical stimulation and free vascularized fibular grafts. Amputation is also a treatment option.

ELECTIVE AMPUTATION AND THE COUPLE RELATIONSHIP

A comprehensive review of the literature indicates that no information exists pertaining to the challenges faced by couples who face the decision regarding elective amputation. Literature does address parental stress toward the physical handicaps of infants and children (e.g., Frey, Greenberg, & Fewell, 1989; Simmons, Fowler & Levison, 1990; Beckman, 1983; Patterson, 1985; Rolland, 1994), long term pediatric illness (e.g., Boll, Dimino, & Matheson, 1978; Holroyd & Guthrie, 1986; Tavormina, Boll, Dunn, Luscomb, & Taylor, 1981) and pediatric terminal illness (e.g., Koch, 1985).

In unfortunate situations where the amputation of an infant's limb is inevitable (e.g., accident, cancer, etc.) parents are left with no alternatives and ruefully follow through on medical advice. Despite the decision appearing straightforward, the stress and anguish experienced by these parents can be enormous. For many, the hopes and dreams they have held for their child are dashed and are quickly replaced by apprehension about his or her present and future well-being. In comparable circumstances that are less straightforward, such as in the case of elective amputation, several salient factors can emerge during the preoperative period that affect the parental decision making process.

THE PREOPERATIVE PERIOD: EMERGING ISSUES AND PARENTAL RESPONSE

Butler, Turkal, and Seidl (1992) address the need for psychological intervention during the preoperative period. Although the information provided by these authors refers specifically to the needs of the patient, the importance of the preoperative period for significant others who may also be profoundly affected during this time is crucial. According to these authors, appropriate preoperative intervention is associated with less complicated postoperative adjustment and grieving.

Although the preoperative period allows the opportunity for psychological preparation (Butler & Turkal, 1992), this time frame can also abound with anxiety and apprehension. As pointed out by Varni and Setoguchi (1993), " . . . parents of children with chronic physical disorders are themselves an at-risk group for psychological adjustment difficulties" (p. 18). Although this clinical data refers to parents of children who have existing chronic physical disorders, it can be hypothesized that parents who envision similar circumstances for their children may also experience personal psychological adjustment problems. Moreover, as personal distress filters down into the couple relationship, established couple patterns can be strained leading to unanticipated intimate and family relationship issues as discussed below.

Boundary Clarification

When various medical options are available to the infant, a couple is introduced to a more complex decision making process which requires careful reflection. Additionally, this often is influenced by internal and external dynamics. For example, in reaction to the news of an infant who is in an unstable medical condition, family members and friends tend to become emotional and protective and try to alleviate parental despair by offering well-intended advice. As more people learn about the couple's unfortunate circumstances, a corresponding curiosity ensues culminating in additional questions.

As advice and questions begin to mount regarding the infant's condition, the couple re-lives their trauma, experiences added stress and often senses a kind of disorientation. In an effort to secure personal space, regain their composure and avoid repetitive responses, the couple may isolate themselves. As a result of their withdrawal, they become further separated from their support network. Varni and Setoguchi (1993) elaborate on the issue of parental social support and a pediatric chronic physical disorder and write, " . . . it is not social connections per se that are protective against psychological maladjustment but rather how the person perceives and interprets his or her social network that determines the protective function of social support" (p. 14). In short, parents can experience a personal *tug-of-war* [italics added] wherein at some level they desire the support of others yet they begin to feel overwhelmed when there is an onslaught of expressed concern. It becomes difficult to ponder conflicting opinions and information and for some, remaining silent about their infant's disorder seems like their only recourse.

Being hesitant to engage others and share their anxiety and worry, the couple typically turns toward each other for support and reassurance. A sudden increase in couple interdependence can contribute to tension, fatigue, and unanticipated conflict. Because each parent is deeply immersed in their infant's medical condition, the couple's conversation inevitably drifts toward medical advice, treatment options, and short and long term implications. As they become engulfed by the details and ramifications of the disorder they find themselves reacting to one another's anxiety. Often, what prevails is lowered tolerance between the couple and increased tension within their relationship.

The decision to withhold information from significant others is rarely straightforward. It becomes further complicated when one partner feels obligated to significant others and opposes any form of social withdrawal or when there are other children involved who express a need to discuss their concerns with extended family members or close friends. Due to the gravity of the situation, rather than serving as active listeners with children, extended family or friends typically react by offering opinions and personal advice. Although a child's request to process new information is normal and appropriate the couple may find themselves with the added duty of having to process superfluous information with their children. During the former scenario, differing individual response patterns or cultural differences that exist between the couple may surface. For instance, if one partner begins to suppress information or avoid discussion regarding the infant's disorder, this behavior may set off a systemic reaction from his or her partner couched in resentment. Often the partner who desires social interaction and disclosure feels as though he or she is left shouldering the burden of explaining, updating, and maintaining outside contact.

There is certainly no one appropriate parental response style to an infant's medical condition. The prevalent view that parents need to share their despair with their social support system is a general recommendation although it is not fitting for all. Pollin (1995) elaborates: "Interpersonal relations are probably the most obvious dimension of family life; family members continuously struggle to maintain intimacy and mutual support. Besides strengthening their communication and coping skills for new challenges, they must reconcile members' differing coping styles and developmental needs and levels" (p. 123).

Case Vignette

Mike and Gail gained confirmation of their infant's CPT following a brief consultation with a surgical resident and pediatric orthopedic surgeon. After hearing the physicians explain that amputation might be a likely outcome, Gail immediately began to visibly express her sorrow through tears. Mike, on the other hand, responded by asking the physicians for clarification and for practical information. Worried about Gail's distraught condition, the surgeon encouraged Mike to console his wife while seemingly ignoring his need for a different kind of support.

Mike's reaction could be considered as a form of denial and/or a lack of attention or concern for his partner. In assuming this perspective, however, individual coping styles are overlooked. Furthermore, inviting an interactional style that contradicts the couple's current functioning style can inadvertently create additional relationship problems.

OUTSIDE INFLUENCES

Although every family situation is unique, several influential groups or figures can impact the decision making process. Couples who are in close proximity to relatives may depend more on the support of family members. In contrast, couples who are not close to family may rely more on the medical profession for support. An overview of the various individuals who are influential during the decision making process follows.

Families-of-Origin

Without question, the reactions of family-of-origin members can significantly impact the couple while they consider the options for their infant. Grandparents, for example, often express concern for their own children, their other grandchildren, as well as the infant. In terms of grandparent reactions, Albrecht (1995) writes:

> Sometimes, their grief makes it difficult for them to be supportive, especially in the beginning. Occasionally, old family conflicts will flare up at this time and you and your spouse may find yourselves listening to old complaints about why you should never have been married in the first place. Sometimes, especially if they are not able to see the child frequently, grandparents refuse to believe anything is really wrong, or cling to the belief that the child will outgrow the disability. (p. 33)

This suggests two problematic reactions from grandparents: one is a form of denial where they respond optimistically and almost dismiss the seriousness of the situation. This reaction can be especially disturbing for couples who are accustomed to turning to their parents to process everyday circumstances and options. Fueled by the hopes and dreams they hold for their grandchild, grandparents may enter into a period of mourning that hinders their ability to be supportive. Couples who have experienced this second problematic response describe how their own parents appeared paralyzed and were seemingly unable to discuss alternatives with them. Not all grandparents or extended family members are unable to provide helpful support. In fact, grandparents can be a tremendous source of strength and support (Rolland, 1994). The purpose of discussing these different responses is to demonstrate the additional stress a couple can experience while having to remain focused on the daily care of the infant, their other children, their relationship, and the inevitable decision they must make.

When issues are left unresolved between the generations, however, a problematic cycle can emerge between grandparents and the biological parents of the infant. This cycle involves the biological parents becoming protective of their own parents by withholding information and any expression of their own grief. In turn, the grandparents pursue the parents for any current medical information. As such, tension can build between the generations and spill over into the couple relationship.

Case Vignette

In response to her daughter's medical condition, Marg became uncharacteristically quiet and emotionally distant from both her parents and her mother and father-in-law. Being known as a mother who would proudly discuss the accomplishments and developmental stages of her children, Marg was behaving in an unusual fashion. Becoming increasingly concerned about his partner's behavioral change, Ted pursued Marg in an effort to determine the source of her sudden behavioral change. Marg perceived Ted's well-intended effort as intrusive and consequently, hostile interactions developed between them.

After taking the opportunity to discuss their growing conflict, Ted learned that Marg perceived her daughter's medical condition as a very personal and private matter. As such, Marg was uncomfortable disclosing what she considered to be highly intimate information.

Medical Community

Different parental experiences and interactions with the medical community result in varying personal accounts. The relationship between the pediatric orthopedic surgeon, family physician and the medical support staff is critical in the decision making process. For couples who feel that their concerns or questions were sidestepped or dismissed, their evaluation of the assistance and direction they received is generally less favorable. Couples who feel that they received the attention they required are more likely to report favorable evaluations.

Due to the complexity and indeterminate nature of the infant's condition, parents can become frustrated with the medical community's inability to provide adequate answers and prognoses. As noted earlier, associated medical conditions further confound the situation.

Professional Reaction

Some couples report that the decision making process also appears to be very difficult for the medical community. Figely (1995) has underscored the stress experienced by professionals who deal with traumas experienced by children. Professionals who appear distant or disengaged may not be demonstrating a disinterest but rather reacting to their own sadness or sense of powerlessness to help the infant and his or her distressed parents. Some physicians may be reluctant to disclose their personal distress with patients due to a perceived threat to the established professional-patient hierarchy. Unfortunately, undisclosed professional distress can be misinterpreted and can lead to unnecessary discomfort and confusion within the professional-family relationship. One couple reported that after sharing their decision to have their infant's leg amputated with the pediatric orthopedic surgeon, the surgeon appeared visibly relieved. This sign of relief could have been due to several factors, including the fact that an ultimate decision had been reached by the parents.

Since CPT is a rare disorder, general practitioners are likely to be unaware of its etiology, prevalence, treatment options, and outcome. The family physician still assumes a central role with families dealing with this condition. Commenting on this role, Butler and Turkal (1992) state, "The family physician can promote patient adjustment by providing accurate information, eliciting unspoken fears, and encouraging the involvement of the patient's family" (p. 69). Unless family physicians are familiar with the complexity of this disorder, its seriousness may not be fully recognized and a false hope can be inferred during the deliberation period.

Case Vignette

During initial physical examinations with their family doctor, Kevin and Susan were reassured that things would *work out fine* [italics added] for their infant son. Because CPT had not yet been diagnosed, the well-intended physician maintained an optimistic attitude and did not allude to any potential problems. In reaction to their physician's reassurance, both Kevin and Susan were relieved to know that many of their worries were most likely unfounded. In fact, the couple recalled a nurse in the delivery room who also suggested that it appeared as though their infant son simply had a dislocated ankle. To the dismay of Kevin and Susan, however, after a scheduled consultation with a pediatric surgeon, the CPT diagnosis was made.

Subjective Perseverance

Physicians who are committed to preserving the infant's limb may suggest to parents that if it were his or her choice as a parent, he or she would favor ongoing surgical intervention (e.g., intramedullary rod, Ilizarov technique) opposed to amputation. Such remarks can further compound and confuse the decision making process for parents, particularly in situations where one parent is in agreement with the surgeon and one parent is not. What generally emerges under these circumstances is a rift within the couple relationship. The spouse who disagrees with the physician's decision perceives his or her partner to be in coalition with the professional and experiences a sense of exclusion or even betrayal. The despondence and vulnerability that parents can experience during the decision making process is profound. Desperately wanting to help their infant, they look to professionals for advice, direction, and support even at the risk of threatening their relationship.

OUT OF THE SPOTLIGHT:
SIBLINGS OF DISABLED CHILDREN

It is natural for people to gravitate to an infant who is in a precarious medical condition. Experiencing sadness for his or her predicament and the hardships that he or she may have to endure, people often express sympathy and a sense of protectiveness. Although this reaction is to be expected, it can have implications for siblings who tend to be overlooked during this process (McKeever, 1983; Rolland, 1994; Schreiber, 1993).

Once the center of attention, siblings often are overshadowed by the special needs of the infant and do not receive the recognition they need. Regardless of the time and energy parents devote to preparing older children for the attention that will be directed toward their younger sibling, the experience of feeling displaced can be very difficult. To prevent sibling jealousy and resentment, parents face the added responsibility of reminding relatives and friends to acknowledge older children despite their immediate concern about the infant. Parents also need to continually debrief these youngsters about the sudden attention bestowed upon their sibling. Although parents run the risk of becoming preoccupied, overwhelmed, and exhausted with their personal circumstances, finding time to listen to their other children's questions and concerns is essential (Albrecht, 1995; Schreiber, 1993). According to Rolland (1994), "Direct and clear information and supportive reassurance from parents are the best preventive medicine for well siblings. Because of embarrassment, conditions that have visible symptoms are usually the most disturbing to siblings" (p. 218).

Case Vignette

Having become accustomed to receiving attention from family friends and relatives prior to the birth of his younger brother who was diagnosed with CPT, Terry began to exhibit inappropriate attention-seeking behaviors whenever he and his family were in the presence of company. Although Terry's parents anticipated some sibling reaction to the birth of their son, they were perplexed by his unprecedented behavior. Upon reflection, Terry's parents began to realize how his presence was diminished by the special circumstances of his brother. They became increasingly aware of the inordinate amount of attention their younger child was receiving.

Helping prepare children for the arrival of a new sibling generally involves ongoing conversations and reassurances about temporary sacrifices and changes in family routine. In the case of an unpredictable medical condition, however, family circumstances tend to be more strained, culminating in intense family interactions. What was anticipated to be a period of family celebration can turn into a period of sorrow. For children with CPT, it is very important that the fragile joint within the infant's leg remain isolated and stable to avoid premature fracturing prior to surgical intervention. Unexpected parental vigilance during this period can alter normal family functioning and interactions.

GENDER ISSUES

The way in which the genders are conditioned by society to respond to stress becomes apparent during infant care. Rolland (1994) remarks that gender roles can become skewed under duress. Goodrich, Rampage, Ellman and Halstead (1988) contend that, "men deny their need to be taken care of so as not to seem weak" (p. 115). If the male partner has been conditioned to be authoritative and to solve the presenting problem, rather than process the underlying feelings of the situation, this can contribute to disharmony within the couple relationship.

Because women are usually identified as the major care giver, the majority of communication is directed toward them. Consequently, they are often the first family member to receive important communication and are left with the task of interpreting vital information to their partners. When information is unclear and/or difficult, a woman can be the recipient of her partner's anger which is usually heightened by his fear and insecurities.

According to some women, when first learning about their infant's diagnosis a sense of guilt and self-blame develops. Because the fetus grew in her body, and feeling responsible for the child's well-being, a woman may somehow experience a sense of accountability for the infant's condition. Bepko and Krestan (1990) contend, "Most women err in the direction of doing too much for a handicapped child because they feel guilty and responsible for the problem" (p. 224). Adding to a sense of personal accountability, these women tend to enter into a self-interrogating mode regarding prenatal care and any possible behavior that could have contributed to the child's condition. To counter self-blame, a parent may also make unrealistic demands on her personal time and energy (Rolland, 1994).

Women often seem comfortable in openly expressing their emotional turmoil and grief. On the other hand, men are encouraged to internalize their sadness and work toward immediate problem resolution. Goodrich et al. (1988) suggest that, " . . . merely listening with empathy does not give a man the sense that he is actively providing anything of value, and furthermore is not a highly developed skill in most men" (p. 124). With the female partner wanting to share and discuss her pain, and the male partner needing to disguise his personal distress, the couple can enter into an interactional process riddled with misunderstandings, unnecessary conflicts, and added relationship problems. A woman may misinterpret her partner's seeming distance or reluctance to engage in conversation about their infant's condition as a lack of interest or concern in her or the child. In actuality, however, the partner may be experiencing tremendous internal turmoil. Unfortunately, these interpersonal transactions often occur during critical times when partners need to support and confer with one another.

Case Vignette

Jim and Betty found themselves quarreling more than usual. What used to be common disagreements that were quickly resolved were now major productions fraught with bickering and insults. During heated arguments, Betty found herself accusing Jim of denial regarding their daughter's circumstances and avoiding any meaningful discussions concerning her condition. In response, Jim would make a snide remark and walk away from Betty. This response would only infuriate Betty who, in turn, would pursue Jim. As the intensity between the couple escalated, the source of the couple's friction was lost. Instead of collaborating and combining their efforts to help each other, the couple experienced an animosity that fueled their conflict.

UNFULFILLED DREAMS

For some parents, the thought of having a child who will be less physically capable than his or her peers can also be devastating. Regardless of their ultimate decision (amputation versus surgical procedures to preserve the limb) parents realize that their child will have special needs that may prevent him or her from performing in specific activities and occupations. In addition, depending on the unique circumstances of the child, traditional family activities may have to be reconsidered or altered. Family beliefs, and the meaning attributed to the infant's circumstances, therefore are critical to couple stability and family well-being (Rolland, 1994).

LOSS AND GRIEF

Since actual death has not occurred, or is not imminent, the constructs of loss and grief that are associated with the amputation can be under-appreciated by parents, siblings, and the couple's support network. Unless feelings of loss and grief are identified, they are rarely articulated. Amputation involves a major loss that must be acknowledged and addressed. Often, however, in an effort to alleviate despair, scenarios that appear more severe are presented to the couple as a point of contrast and hope. People in the couple's support network or from the medical or helping professions may go as far as reporting cases where children have excelled after overcoming tremendous adversity. Although well-intended, rather than providing a context wherein the couple can process their emotions, inadvertent efforts are made to solace the couple.

Research conducted by Varni and Setoguchi (1993) considered the effects of parental adjustment on the adaptation of children with congenital or acquired limb deficiencies. Although this particular study pertains to parents with older children who were between the age of eight and 13 years, their findings nevertheless demonstrate the contextual importance of parental response and the emotional disposition of disabled children. These authors report, ". . . based on the extant literature, it would appear that both maternal and paternal emotional distress be considered risk factors for child maladjustment. The findings on marital discord are clear and consistent: higher marital discord statistically predicts higher child depressive symptomatology and trait anxiety and lower general self-esteem, regardless of whether it is paternal or maternal perception of marital functioning" (p. 17).

Grieving Process

The grieving process seems to occur at two distinct levels: the pre-amputation process and the post-amputation process. For the purpose of this paper, the former process will be discussed.

When first learning that their infant has congenital pseudarthrosis, the couple begins to mourn for the child. Although not having yet decided on a medical direction, after the initial consultation with the pediatric surgeon, the couple begins to comprehend the short and long term ramifications of this rare disorder. Realizing that the infant's first few months will not be as expected, and that potential problems may develop, contributes to an aura of sorrow.

In an effort to protect her spouse (and perhaps other children) from additional worry, the woman may choose to express her grief privately. As such, she perceives her grieving as an individual process which needs to occur in isolation. What remains, however, is an uncertainty regarding how to share her despair with her partner. A resentment toward her partner can slowly evolve when the woman feels an increasing need to express her sorrow to her partner but is reluctant to do so. Consequently, the woman begins to feel emotionally distant from her partner while simultaneously concerned about the welfare of her infant.

RECOMMENDATIONS

It appears that couples who find themselves at the crossroads regarding their infant's welfare face the dual task of maintaining a stable relationship while considering the best course of action for their infant. In order to help couples accomplish these tasks, various recommendations are suggested and discussed directly below.

1. In order to gain a clear understanding of their infant's predicament and surgical options, parents can request a comprehensive literature search. To obtain current literature regarding CPT, the couple can elicit the support of their physician. With appropriate literature, the couple can review the current data, become properly informed, and consult with the orthopedic surgeon. Becoming familiar with the available literature can be an empowering experience for the couple during the decision making process. In essence, CPT becomes demystified and the couple can collaborate together and with the health care professional during the learning process. Rather than being pulled apart during their deliberation process, the couple subsystem becomes strengthened and unified.
2. Regardless of their established interactional pattern, the couple can anticipate elevated anxiety, fatigue, and stress. These factors can contribute to unanticipated conflict within their intimate and parental relationship. Predicting challenging and stressful moments can

be a useful way of evading unnecessary hostility and in fact can bolster the couple relationship as they combine forces.

3. Candidly discussing the need for clear boundaries with significant others can also prevent hurt feelings and misunderstandings. When establishing clear boundaries, the couple can describe how they would like to share information and obtain advice. With a preferred method in place, the couple can maintain their social support network without the fear of becoming overwhelmed with suggestions and advice.

4. As a way of coping with personal stress and safeguarding their relationship, the couple can develop and institute personal time-outs. Planned time away from each other, as well as time alone together, can provide the couple with the necessary space to reflect on their experience as individuals and as a couple.

5. Participation in a support group may be helpful. Becoming involved in such a group provides the couple with an opportunity to meet other parents who are facing, or who have faced, similar circumstances, decisions, and challenges.

6. The couple and their other children can also observe youngsters who have either had an amputation, or alternative surgical procedures, while at play. It is not uncommon for parents and siblings to fear that the physically challenged child will be unable to play and enjoy many childhood activities. After observing children, many of these fears can be dispelled.

7. It is important that the couple inform helping professionals of their individual needs. Each family circumstance is unique, and therefore generalizations need to be avoided. Forming a positive relationship with helping professionals can ease the concern of the couple and can be helpful during critical stages of infant care.

CONCLUSION

When a couple is confronted with major medical decisions regarding their infant, unanticipated elevated levels of anxiety and distress can surface. Despite normal effective coping skills, the deliberation process can be highly charged and is rarely straightforward. This paper discussed congenital pseudarthrosis, surgical alternatives that are available to the infant, and the inherent challenges that couples encounter during the decision making process. Particular attention is rendered to the intrapsychic, interpersonal and ecological factors that typically influence the couple relationship during the deliberation process.

Due to the magnitude of their infant's medical condition, a couple may experience a period of disorientation and therefore find themselves despondent and vulnerable. In order to protect their relationship, and avoid unnecessary conflict that can emerge due to fatigue and uncertainty, several practical recommendations have been suggested.

REFERENCES

Albrecht, D. (1995). *Raising a child who has a physical disability.* New York: Wiley.

Apley, J., Barbour, R., & Westmacom, F. (1967). Impact of congenital heart disease on the family: A preliminary report. *British Medical Journal, 1,* 103-105.

Bepko, C. & Krestan, J. (1990). *Too good for her own good: Searching for self and intimacy in important relationships.* New York: Harper Perennial.

Boll, T., Dimino, E., & Matheson, A. (1978). Parenting attitudes: The role of personality style and childhood long-term illness. *Journal of Psychosomatic Research, 22,* 209-213.

Butler, D., Turkal, N., & Seidl, J. (1992). Amputation: Preoperative psychological preparation. *Journal of the American Board of Family Practice, 5,* 69-73.

Figely, C. (1995). Compassion fatigue as a secondary traumatic stress disorder. An overview. In C. Figely (Ed.), *Compassion fatigue: Coping with secondary traumatic stress disorder in those who treat the traumatized.* New York: Brunner/Mazel.

Goodrich, T., Rampage, C., Ellman, B., & Halstead, K. (1988). *Feminist family therapy: A casebook.* New York: Norton.

Holroyd, J., & Guthrie, D. (1986). Family stress with chronic childhood disease: cystic fibrosis neuromuscular disease and renal disease. *Journal of Clinical Psychology, 42,* 552-561.

Lavigne, J., & Ryan, M. (1979). Psychologic adjustment of siblings and children with chronic illness. *Pediatrics, 63,* 616-626.

Linde, L., Rasof, B., & Dunn, O. (1970). Longitudinal studies of intellectual and behavioral development in children with congenital heart disease. *Paediatrica Scandinavia, 59,* 169-176.

McKeever, P. (1983). Siblings of chronically ill children: A literature review with implications for research and practice. *American Journal of Orthopsychiatry, 53,* 209-218.

Pollin, I. (1995). *Medical crisis counseling: Short-term therapy for long-term illness.* New York: Norton.

Rolland, J. (1994). *Families, illness, and disability: An integrative treatment model.* New York: Basic Books.

Schreiber, M. (1993). Forgotten children. In S. Klein and M. Schleifer (Eds.), *It isn't fair! Siblings of children with disabilities* (pp. 33-40). Connecticut: Bergin & Garvey.

Tavormina, B., Boll, T., Luscomb, R., & Taylor, R. (1981). Psychosocial effects on parents raising a physically handicapped child. *Journal of Abnormal Child Psychology, 9,* 121-131.

Varni, J., & Setoguchi, Y. (1993). Effects of parental adjustment on the adaptation of children with congenital or acquired limb deficiencies. *Journal of Developmental and Behavioral Pediatrics, 14,* 13-20.

Intimacy in the Face of Catastrophic Illness

Penny Cupp

SUMMARY. This is a therapist's story of her battle with life-threatening breast cancer and the impact of that illness on the intimacy bond with her husband of thirty years. She reviews the year of treatment, noting the couple's connections at various points in the process of dealing with the disease: the diagnosis, the treatment and the aftermath. Facing life-threatening illness can drive a couple apart or draw them closer together, but whichever it does, it is a loss of innocence about the very real presence of death and its impact on our daily life in relationship. *[Article copies available for a fee from The Haworth Document Delivery Service: 1-800-342-9678. E-mail address: getinfo@ haworthpressinc.com]*

"You have cancer." A sentence we all dread hearing. I was totally unprepared for this news when it was delivered in August, 1995. I had been in excellent health for most of my 47 years, and there was no history of cancer in my family. As a therapist with a special interest in holistic health and stress-related disorders, I had been living my life with an acute awareness of the dangers of Type-A behavior and I ate, exercised, meditated, and worked with a view toward keeping my life balanced to avoid the heart disease which had struck my father at age 38 and killed him at age 58. I had been fighting the wrong disease!

The diagnostic process was very rapid and very frightening. In the course of a single day I saw my primary physician, a breast surgeon and an

---

Penny Cupp, PhD, 5180 Roswell Road N.W., Suite 201 North, Atlanta, GA 30342.

[Haworth co-indexing entry note]: "Intimacy in the Face of Catastrophic Illness." Cupp, Penny. Co-published simultaneously in *Journal of Couples Therapy* (The Haworth Press, Inc.) Vol. 7, No. 4, 1998, pp. 63-67; and: *Couples, Trauma, and Catastrophes* (ed: Barbara Jo Brothers) The Haworth Press, Inc., 1998, pp. 63-67. Single or multiple copies of this article are available for a fee from The Haworth Document Delivery Service [1-800-342-9678, 9:00 a.m. - 5:00 p.m. (EST). E-mail address: getinfo@ haworthpressinc.com].

© 1998 by The Haworth Press, Inc. All rights reserved.

oncologist. I had regular mammograms and had one just six months earlier. While on vacation, I had noticed a curious red patch on the skin of my left breast. When I went in to see my primary physician, she wanted me to see a surgeon and the one she recommended had a cancellation that afternoon. He took one look at the redness and said "You have inflammatory breast cancer." Biopsy results would later confirm the diagnosis. He called an oncologist whom he respected. Dr. D. had just left for the day–it was 3:00 on Friday afternoon, but his secretary caught him on the car phone. He came back to his office and spent two hours with me, explaining my diagnosis, prognosis, and treatment recommendations. Because of the aggressiveness of this type of cancer (fifteen years ago the 2-year survival rate was zero) he felt there was not a minute to lose in starting treatment.

I remember thinking as I left his office that I was glad that I was by myself. Being alone with the doctors and the news forced me to focus, in spite of my shock, on hearing what they were saying to me. If my husband, Lloyd, had been with me I think I would have had the luxury of falling apart. I needed some time to digest this news before I could talk about it with anyone.

When I got home that evening, I greeted Lloyd with a hug and said something like, "We've got some serious talking to do. I have cancer." In the 29 years of our marriage, this was probably the biggest test of the intimacy bond between us. Rather than driving a wedge in our connection, it drew a silver cord around us, pulling us close together in our pain and fear. We had been through many stages of marital development and many crises of living. Each of us has lost a father and a brother and Lloyd has lost his mother, as well. But this ultimate crisis, the threat of one of our deaths and permanent separation, was not supposed to come along for several years yet. We cried together, held each other, told our children, family and friends.

In the literature on stress and coping, it is commonly acknowledged that a person's ability to withstand stress is directly related to the strength of his or her coping resources. I think this is true for couples as well. We had so many resources to draw on: our own spiritual beliefs, an optimistic attitude toward life, the depth of our connection that had survived many trials, a terrific support network among family and friends, and a medical team that was not only knowledgeable, but also caring and respectful of us as persons. Somewhere I read that half of the women who lose a breast to cancer also lose a mate. It would be interesting to know whether that is because the partner could not handle the intense feelings occasioned by illness, grief and loss, or because the woman herself decided that the relationship was somehow inhibiting her health and growth as a person. Whatever the reason, the intimacy bond had failed. There's a great research study in there somewhere.

In the weeks and months that followed, our bond was tested again and again. When you think you, or your spouse, is going to die, it rearranges your priorities in a hurry. The little things that bug you about your partner—and even many of the big things—just seem to evaporate as inconsequential. Our initial response to this catastrophic illness was to be very loving and very kind to each other. But that becomes harder to do as time and treatment wear on.

I remember one evening about a month after I began treatment I had an outpatient surgery to confirm the diagnosis and to implant a catheter in my chest wall through which they would administer the chemotherapy. I had two infusions of chemo, my hair had all fallen out, and I had to learn to give myself injections to boost my sagging white blood count. Lloyd was looking at the pitiful sight that was me with tears in his eyes. I said, "Come on, we haven't even gotten to the hard parts yet." He said, "Penny, they're all hard parts."

In the weeks that followed we talked about the things that I suppose all couples should talk about but probably don't. We talked about my dying, where and how I wanted to by buried, how I hoped his life would be without me. Those are hard parts, too. I think of intimacy as occurring at three different levels. At level one you talk about things, other people, opinions, situations that affect you. At level two you talk about your *feelings* about things, people, opinions, and situations. At level three, you talk about your deepest feelings about each other and the relationship you have. We were definitely covering all the levels.

Of course we did not maintain this intensity all the time. Even within the limitations of the illness we found ways to play, ways to laugh, ways to be with other people. And we drifted onto times of separation and loneliness.

Around the time of my surgery, three months after treatment began, I was aware of drawing women around me to be with me in my healing. I was particularly dependent on my daughter Amy, a beautiful young adult who is also an old soul, my sister Pam, and my women friends. I think Lloyd began to feel shut out of my healing circle. But I knew that these women had something to give me that I needed, something that Lloyd couldn't give. They understood at a level he (and no other man) could ever understand about what it meant to be losing my breast. Lloyd was there, but more on the periphery. And I think he resented that he had less access to me, and also felt terribly helpless to do anything. And "doing something" is so much a part of a man's make-up. I think that was also a problem for my son Trey; living a thousand miles away added to his feelings of helplessness.

In February, 1996, I was coming to the end of chemotherapy and had pretty well recovered from a modified radical mastectomy in November. I was about to embark on the third leg of treatment, which was radiation. I could see a light at the end of the tunnel. Then my doctor introduced a detour. He recommended that I undergo high dose chemotherapy (HDC) and bone marrow transplant (BMT). After consultations and second opinions we decided that this was my best chance for long-term survival and agreed to the procedure. Without the transplant I had about a 40% chance of survival at two years after diagnosis. With the transplant the probability of disease-free survival is 70% at five years. It seemed worth the risk. We'd been through lots of hard parts, but this was, without a doubt, the hardest.

To describe the procedure as briefly as I can, HDC/BMT is a process of extracting some healthy bone marrow and freezing it, administering potentially lethal doses of chemotherapy which take white blood and platelet counts down to zero, and then "rescuing" the patient by re-introduction of the frozen marrow. The day of implanting the healthy marrow is referred to as your "new birthday," because the process takes you to the edge of death and then brings you back. My "new birthday" is May 20, 1996.

I was in the hospital for three and a half weeks. I had been stripped of my hair and my breast, but the bone marrow procedure stripped me of even deeper parts of what had made me who I am. I have almost no memories of the hospital stay. High doses of morphine and ativan are responsible for that. I lost my entire immune system, my strength, my energy, even the inflections in my voice. I lost my sexuality. I lost my taste for alcohol, coffee, and carbonated drinks. I lost my sense of time and space. I lost my life and was brought back. Some members of my family was with me the entire time, because I knew I would not be able to be present for myself. I needed a loving presence and they were there.

In the weeks after I came home, I went through the dying process in reverse, or perhaps it was re-birth. I could hardly walk or talk in the early days. I gradually reclaimed most of what I had lost. Thanks to plastic surgery I have a new "breast" and a flat tummy; my hair is growing back with a lot more gray than I remember. My energy is back; I drink coffee and an occasional glass of wine. Next summer we'll see if I need to be re-immunized for all the childhood diseases. I am oriented × 3. One of the lessons of cancer is that time is the most precious thing we have. I hope that's something I don't forget as I become well and strong again. Because of the synchonicity of timing, Lloyd, who is a school teacher, was on summer vacation during my convalescence and we were able to be together constantly during my recovery.

Last year, shortly after my diagnosis, I was doing a lot of reading and listening to tapes to try to make sense of what was happening to me, and to us. I read/heard in several different places that some people feel like cancer was the best thing that ever happened to them. I certainly could not say that, then or now. Cancer is a terrible disease. But I began to think about what I would list as the "best things" that have ever happened to me. Marrying Lloyd would certainly be on that list, as well as the births of our two children. Becoming a therapist is one of the best things that ever happened to me. People and connections, rather than events, seem to characterize my "best things." I realize that having cancer does have some things in common with my "best things." None of the best things were about pure bliss. Each was a context which produced profound growth and challenge and change. Each of those events set the stage for a deeper experience of pain and joy, hope and despair, inviting–no, demanding of me a deeper engagement with myself and others in the process of defining self and relationships. The best things that ever happened to me have been those moments of authentic connection between my most real self and that of another person. That is worth struggling for, worth risking the pain that is inevitably tied to intimacy.

As I reclaim myself and restructure my new life, we are also exploring new ways of relating. Cancer has made me more honest, less willing to accommodate and wait my turn. I want connection and I want it now! We both still have many strong feelings that we are continuing to work through, together and separately. We learned about "in sickness and in health" at a new level. We take nothing for granted anymore; there was a loss of innocence in facing this cancer. One of us will die first, leaving the other alone. We are weaving new threads, as fine and as strong as a spider's web, into our intimacy bond, so that it can withstand the next onslaught, whatever that might be. And when it comes, we will face it together.

The Negative Impact
of Survivor Guilt on Marriage

Richard Vogel

SUMMARY. Individuals who grow up with self-denying and/or unhappy parents or siblings often develop pathogenic beliefs that prevent them from enjoying themselves or their relationships. Unconscious beliefs emanating from survivor guilt in relation to individuals who are not faring as well as oneself occasion maladaptive behaviors, i.e., undoing, unprovoked antagonism, withdrawal, that are harmful to a marriage. By behaving in this manner, individuals susceptible to the effects of survivor guilt are unwittingly maintaining loyalty to their unhappy parent(s) or sibling(s), at the price of their own happiness. *[Article copies available for a fee from The Haworth Document Delivery Service: 1-800-342-9678. E-mail address: getinfo@ haworthpressinc.com]*

Marriages with the potential for growth and continued enrichment are often undermined when partners chronically re-enact with one another maladaptive behaviors acquired in childhood in their relations with unhappy and/or self-denying parents or siblings. The likelihood for such reenactment to occur is magnified to the extent that either or both partners are burdened with unconscious guilt associated with a potential for success in their relationship that was either imperceptible or nonexistent in their parents' relationship and/or unobtainable by their siblings. Such individuals often harbor the unconscious belief that to be successful in their rela-

Richard Vogel, PhD, is a Member of San Francisco Psychotherapy Research Group, 377 Highland Avenue, San Rafael, CA 94901.

[Haworth co-indexing entry note]: "The Negative Impact of Survivor Guilt on Marriage." Vogel, Richard. Co-published simultaneously in *Journal of Couples Therapy* (The Haworth Press, Inc.) Vol. 7, No. 4, 1998, pp. 69-79; and: *Couples, Trauma, and Catastrophes* (ed: Barbara Jo Brothers) The Haworth Press, Inc., 1998, pp. 69-79. Single or multiple copies of this article are available for a fee from The Haworth Document Delivery Service [1-800-342-9678, 9:00 a.m. - 5:00 p.m. (EST). E-mail address: getinfo@haworthpressinc.com].

© 1998 by The Haworth Press, Inc. All rights reserved.

tionship is to demonstrate disloyalty and possibly harm their less fortunate parents or siblings.

The concept of survivor guilt was introduced by Niederland (1981) who described a persevering guilt complex affecting survivors of the Holocaust. Survivors developed symptoms that included depression, anhedonia, psychosomatic conditions and anxiety. Niederland viewed these symptoms as identifications with family members who had not survived and ascribed them a pervasive and intense sense of guilt that he referred to as survivor guilt. Modell (1971) states that survivor guilt is based upon the belief that taking is at someone else's expense. According to Modell, survivor guilt stems from a biologically-based concern for and sensitivity to the pain of significant others, making it difficult to be happy if others are not.

Weiss and Sampson (1986) use the term "survivor guilt" to connote the guilt of persons who assume they have fared better than their parents or siblings. A person experiencing the debilitating effects of survivor guilt believes, according to Weiss and Sampson, that "by acquiring more of the good things of life than parents or siblings, he has betrayed them. . . . His acquisitions have been obtained at the expense of parents or siblings" (p. 52).

In a similar vein, Firestone (1987), in his book, *The Fantasy Bond*, comments:

> Guilt in relation to other people who are self-denying takes the joy out of achievement . . . most people unconsciously deprive themselves of much of what they value in life because they fear going beyond a significant person in their background. (p. 229)

Engel and Ferguson (1990) elaborate on the implication of "outdoing," i.e., surpassing, a family member. According to Engel and Ferguson (1990) "the crime of outdoing" stems from two irrational beliefs. (1) ". . . by having the good things in life (happiness, success, love and affection) you are using them up, not leaving any for your less fortunate parents or siblings." (2) ". . . by achieving your occupational and personal goals, you are showing up those family members who were unable to achieve their own" (p. 42).

In the novel *The Prince of Tides* (Conroy, 1991), Tom's moodiness and rejection of his wife's affection are manifestations of survivor guilt associated with his brother's violent death and his sister's incarceration in a mental hospital. In response to her husband's despondency, self-deprecation and the effect his moods are having on her, Tom's wife, Sally, implores him to give up his sorrowful ways and be more demonstratively affectionate. She remarks "You've been so self-pitying, so analytical and so bitter, since what happened to Luke. You've got to forget what happened and go on from here, from this moment. Your life isn't over, Tom. . . . Why do you want to throw even the good things away?" (p. 26). Tom's hopelessness is evident in his response "Because they aren't so good to me anymore, because I don't believe in my life anymore" (p. 27). This is the voice of his survivor guilt speaking and echoes his refusal to acquiesce to his wife's invitation to a happier life. He simply cannot allow himself pleasure in the wake of his siblings' tragic lives.

With regards to the detrimental effects of survivor guilt, Firestone (1988) comments:

> The person who is alive to his experience may unconsciously hold back his enthusiasm, sensing that his vitality might threaten a person who is more self-denying . . . we have observed that people are very susceptible to negative social pressure from unhappy or self-sacrificing family members. (p. 266)

CLINICAL CASE EXAMPLES

A dramatic example whereby a marriage with the potential for success was placed at risk as a result of one of the partners feeling obligated to his unhappy and visibly distraught mother occurred as follows: Ben, his wife and widowed mother were viewing a film in which a couple were passionately embracing. Ben's mother, peering intently at her son with the glint of an all-too-familiar carefully contrived tear in her eye, lamented "I wish I had some of that."

In couples therapy, Ben's therapist inquired whether his mother's despairing comment had affected him. He replied that it had not, but admitted that he had became embroiled in a bitter fight with his wife, jealous that she had spent the evening with her girlfriends.

Ben learned to be possessive in relation to his mother, who had been extremely needy and demanding of her son's attention throughout his childhood. This tendency was exacerbated after the death of her husband, when Ben became her sole source of affection.

Ben harbored the pathogenic belief (Weiss, 1993), fueled by his mother's neediness and poverty of relationships, that it was his responsibility to make her happy. The impossibility of doing so, combined with his mother's obvious despair, engendered intense guilt for Ben. According to Weiss (1993):

A person develops pathogenic beliefs in childhood by inferring them from traumatic experiences with parents and siblings. These are experiences in which he finds that by attempting to attain a normal, desirable goal, he brings about a disruption in his ties to his parents. For example, he may infer that he burdens his parents by being dependent on them, or that he causes them to feel hurt and rejected by being independent of them. (p. 6)

Ben assuaged his guilt by providing the appearance of not being any more happy in his life than his mother was in hers. He accomplished this grim result by adopting the worst of his mother's traits, her possessiveness which he inflicted upon his well-meaning spouse.

It is often the case that instead of rejecting parental attitudes and behaviors detrimental to their happiness, individuals like Ben adopt and reenact these very same attributes. By maintaining their allegiance with their parents' shortcomings, they are in some obscure fashion magically protecting and providing redemption for their parents' flawed personalities. Fishel (1991), in her book *Family Mirrors*, elaborates upon this phenomenon as follows:

... From childhood forward we will make a huge effort to prove our parents right, even if it means making ourselves wrong. ... we may maintain our childhood loyalty to our parents by continuing the ... abuse, ensuring that we will not outdo our parents as parents. (p. 84)

According to Weiss and Sampson (1986), individuals like Ben who are susceptible to survivor guilt inflict punishment on themselves to atone for their attainment of a more prosperous existence than their despondent parent.

He may by identifying with the parent towards whom he feels guilty acquire certain of the parents most self-destructive behaviors or traits . . . for example ruin his marriage by raging at his wife as his father ruined his marriage by such raging. (p. 51)

Ben experienced his wife's anger in response to his possessiveness, as punishment for being in a relationship with her that afforded him happiness, and that contrasted so dramatically with his mother's despair.

When this dynamic was discussed in therapy, Ben was able to gain insight into the disruptive effects to his marriage of his possessiveness. This awareness enabled him to resist the temptation to compensate for his mother's unhappiness through the enactment of undermining behaviors that placed his marriage in jeopardy.

Another instance where the presence of survivor guilt was injurious to a marriage occurred for Jack, a writer, at the time of the publication of his first novel. Simultaneously, with its publication, Jack visited his younger brother who was in the throes of coping with two crises–a divorce and the loss of his job. Though Jack was consciously aware of the sadness he felt for his brother's hardship, he was ill-prepared for what would eventually manifest as a self-denying symptomatic expression of his concern. This took the form of his experiencing erection dysfunction after the visit.

Apparently, Jack's achievement juxtaposed with his brother's recent business failure and divorce engendered guilt that negatively affected his relationship with his wife, depriving him of what had been an exciting and spirited sexual relationship.

Firestone (1988) comments on this dynamic as follows:

> . . . achievement, an unusual success, or personal fulfillment in a relationship often lead to anxiety states that precipitate withholding responses. . . . Patterns of withholding practiced by one partner can effectively change the other's positive feelings of love to those of hostility and anger. For example, men and women often hold back qualities that originally attracted their mates, such as their . . . sexual involvement. (p. 169)

Jack's erection dysfunction and the conflict it created between him and his wife evened the score for outdoing his brother in the domains of work and love. Though he had received accolades for his novel, he nevertheless found himself in the less-than-enviable position of a discordant relationship with his wife that mirrored his brother's inharmonious marriage.

Though Jack consciously desired to enjoy the fruits of his literary endeavors along with an intimate relationship with his wife, his unconscious guilt and the belief that he was unentitled to success while his brother's life was in such turmoil prevented him from doing so.

One aim of the couples therapy was to enhance Jack's awareness of the origins of his grim belief while receiving encouragement from both his wife and myself to overcome its implications. Such an awareness would enable Jack to challenge this belief, regain his sexual vigor and attain a level of satisfaction in his marriage that had been available to him prior to visiting his brother. Upon his return I asked Jack how he felt about his brother's divorce and loss of his job. Jack said that he was "saddened" by these events. He lamented how his mood had changed from one of elation associated with the publication of his novel, to despair in relation to his brother's dilemma. Jack shared a dream indicative of his guilt and fear of surpassing his brother. In his dream, Jack portrayed his brother as a prestigious CEO of a large corporation, a far cry from his current unemployed status. Jack interpreted his dream as a wish to elevate his brother in stature to compensate for his recent losses. I observed that Jack might be feeling guilty regarding his brother's difficult straits at a time when Jack was experiencing success as a novelist. In response to my interpretation, Jack recalled having similar feelings upon graduating from college with honors while concurrently his brother was graduating from high school with no plans to continue his education. After that event, Jack "never felt right" discussing his achievements with his brother for fear of "showing him up" and/or "hurting his feelings," an earlier manifestation of Jack's survivor guilt. His wife concurred that on numerous occasions she observed Jack minimize his accomplishments in conversations with his brother. Jack utilized his wife's and his therapist's observations to refute his pathogenic belief that his achievements were potentially harmful to his brother.

In an attempt to remedy his erection dysfunction, a symptomatic manifestation of his survivor guilt, Jack requested that he and his wife go on a date and that upon their return, his wife wear a negligee that he had given her to celebrate their anniversary. Jack was confident that with his newly-acquired insights, regarding the role of survivor guilt in his life, combined with a more novel approach to their sexuality, that his sexual difficulties would subside. Jack's wife was delighted with her husband's change in attitude and in subsequent sessions reported having achieved intercourse devoid of any complications.

Altruistic attempts like Jack's to compensate for the despair and unhappiness of loved ones by suffering in kind are doomed to fail. Yet such behaviors occur frequently in the lives of men and women.

A married couple on their honeymoon received a frantic call from the bride's mother who was experiencing an attack of vertigo. Each day of the honeymoon, and much to her husband's chagrin, Rachel, the bride, though desirous of distancing herself from her mother, was motivated by guilt to call her. To atone for the guilt induced by her mother's insinuation that she was neglecting her, she deprived herself of her husband's affection and good will. Rachel's guilt for daring to enjoy her life with her husband, while her mother manifested such intense though contrived suffering, required that she subvert her good intentions towards him.

Rheingold (1964) counsels women in Rachel's situation as follows:

> A woman may bring any number of assets to marriage—compassion, wisdom, intelligence, skills, an imaginative spirit, delight-giving femininity, good humor, friendliness, pride in a job well done—but if she does not bring emancipation from her mother, the assets may

wither or may be overbalanced by the liability of the fear of being a woman. (p. 451)

In couples therapy, I asked Rachel how she felt about her mother's interference at a time when Rachel should have been accorded the opportunity to celebrate her marriage. Rachel replied that for as long as she remembered, her mother had behaved selfishly towards her, placing her voracious need for attention above her daughter's right to a life independent of such manipulation. Rachel recalled depriving herself of friends, hobbies and a close relationship with her father in response to her mother's incessant plea for her daughter's undivided attention. She described her mother as a needy, unhappy woman who rather than create a life for herself, was living vicariously through her daughter.

Rachel's husband reported numerous incidents where his mother-in-law attempted to subvert their marriage. He believed that Rachel's mother would be happy with him out of the picture. Rachel understood that by succumbing to her mother's selfish and unreasonable demands, she would be placing her marriage in jeopardy.

On one occasion Rachel posed an unconscious test (Weiss and Sampson, 1986) for her therapist. The purpose of this test was to disconfirm her pathogenic belief acquired in relation to her mother that her autonomous strivings were injurious to others. According to Weiss and Sampson unconscious testing of the therapist is a means by which patients attempt to solve their problems. By provoking the therapist and monitoring his response, the patient is able to determine whether certain of his unconscious beliefs are really true.

Engel and Ferguson (1990) describe the "transference test" as one in which:

> the client invites or provokes the therapist to treat him in the same negative way that he was treated by his parents. If the parent was critical, the client invites the therapist to be critical. If the parent was controlling, the client invites the therapist to be controlling . . . to pass these tests, the therapist must refuse these invitations. (p. 202)

According to Engel and Ferguson (1990), what the patient unconsciously desires "is for the therapist to demonstrate that he will not criticize her, or control her-even if given the opportunity" thus allowing her to "overcome her unconscious beliefs that she deserves these inequities" (p. 203).

Rachel's test took the form of her announcing her intention to enter a week-long couples' retreat as an adjunct to her couples therapy. Unlike her mother who denied and denigrated her daughter's attempts at individuating, I encouraged Rachel to proceed with her plan agreeing that it would be useful to her marriage. According to Weiss and Sampson (1986), when a test is passed:

> the patient may become unconsciously less anxious and more relaxed than he had been. He may, moreover, while relaxed, become more insightful. He may, for example, bring forth a previously repressed memory. . . . He may, in addition, keep the memory in consciousness without coming into conflict with it and use the insight he gained from it to attain a better understanding of his problems. (p. 106)

In a subsequent session, Rachel vividly recalled the childhood experience of being denied access to a ballet class by her mother, who chided Rachel for being "too chubby" to succeed in such an endeavor. Rachel felt relieved that I, unlike her mother, responded to her attempts at individuation non-punitively and with encouragement. Rachel's husband added that by supporting Rachel's independent strivings, I had provided him with role modeling that he intended to replicate on those occasions when he, like Rachel's mother, tended to be critical of his wife.

Rachel's awareness of the dynamics underlying her relationship with her mother, combined with her therapist's passing of her transference test, provided Rachel with the motivation to challenge and overcome her belief that her autonomous strivings were harmful to others. This enabled her to affiliate more comfortably with her husband and resist the temptation to experience intimacy in their relationship as a disloyalty to her mother.

Wallerstein and Blakeslee (1995), in their book *The Good Marriage*, cautions that for a marriage to flourish, partners are required to separate psychologically from their families' "emotional ties." They write:

> Psychological separation means gradually detaching from your family's emotional ties . . . you must shift your primary love and loyalty to the marital partner . . . (p. 53). Separation is particularly tricky for women because the ties between mother and daughter, made up of strands of compassion, love, and sometimes guilt, are so powerful . . . Marriage may be particularly hard for the daughter whose mother is lonely and unhappy or is caring for an ill sibling or spouse. (p. 55)

Janet and Lewis entered couples therapy feuding about Janet's perception of her husband's parenting their newborn. On one occasion Lew, upset by their child's continuous crying, cursed out loud and, in Janet's perception, held their infant too tightly while changing diapers. Janet accused her husband of being insensitive. She implied that his outburst and manner of handling their child bordered on being abusive. During our first couples session, Janet intimated that she was considering divorcing her husband. Lew acknowledged that his behavior was out of line, apologized and promised to refrain from reenacting such behavior in the future.

Janet disregarded her husband's apology. She continued to berate him throughout the days that followed. In the interest of defusing their feud, their therapist interpreted Janet's reaction as exemplary of her maternal instinct to protect their infant. Lew responded positively to this interpretation. He viewed Janet as a compassionate, caring woman, character traits that were influential in his decision to marry her. At the same time he remarked how difficult it had been for him to be repeatedly accused of abusing their child, and that no matter what he did to rectify his error, Janet's rancor did not diminish.

Lew contended that this one occasion where he appeared to be losing control was an anomaly. He prided himself on being impeccably attuned to his child's needs. Janet acknowledged Lew's overall sensitivity to their child. Janet surmised that perhaps there might be other factors contributing to her exaggerated response.

Interactions with family members, friends and acquaintances affect one's relationship. Janet's sister, who could not have children, had been visiting at the time this episode took place.

In his book *Voice Therapy*, Firestone (1988) refers to the deleterious effect of guilt activated in proximity to or induced by one's less fortunate and/or envious family members.

> Many patients . . . regress when they have contact with original family members particularly if members of their family either actually manipulate them to activate their guilt feelings or indirectly foster guilt in the patient because of the negative quality of the family members' lives. (p. 229)

Janet felt guilty for being able to conceive a child while her sister could not. Her sister's complaint that Janet had "all the luck" made it even more difficult for Janet to talk about the pleasure she received from her infant. Janet was aware of subduing her feelings and expressions of enthusiasm in relation to her child while in her sister's presence. She remained unaware, however, of the insidious affect to her marriage that her sister's forlorn attitude was creating. Juxtaposed with her good fortune, her sister's unhappiness became the seeds of an inner discontent that would eventually manifest as an overreaction to her husband's relatively benign and remediable error.

The presence of unconscious guilt for surpassing a loved one or attaining in life what they were unable to often manifests as self-sabotaging behavior on the part of the more fortunate individual. Janet's bickering with her husband was meant to convey to her less fortunate sibling that though she appeared to be happier and the recipient of more good fortune, this was not really the case as evidenced in her marital conflict.

Janet's cognizance of her guilt enabled her to communicate her feelings in a more even tempered manner. She viewed her husband as an ally in possession of parenting skills conducive to their child's well being. Rather than divorce, she was determined to react more reasonably to disagreements that invariably arise in the course of child-rearing.

Adolf Guggenbuhl-Craig (1981), in his book *Marriage Dead or Alive*, alludes to the value of persevering and remaining in one's relationship while resisting the temptation to flee when the going gets rough.

> The life-long dialectical encounter between two partners, the bond of man and woman until death, can be understood as a special path for discovering the soul, as a special form of individuation. One of the essential features of this soteriological pathway is the absence of avenues for escape. Just as the saintly hermits cannot evade themselves, so the married persons cannot avoid their partners. In this partially uplifting, partially tormenting evasionlessness lies the specific character of this path. (p. 41)

REFERENCES

Conroy, P. (1991). *The prince of tides*. New York: Bantam Books.

Engel, L. & Ferguson, T. (1990). *Imaginary crimes*. Boston: Houghton Mifflin Company.

Firestone, R.W. (1987). *The fantasy bond*. Los Angeles, CA: Human Sciences Press.

Firestone, R.W. (1988). *Voice therapy*. New York: Human Sciences Press.

Fishel, E. (1991). *Family mirrors*. Boston: Houghton Mifflin Company.

Guggenbuhl-Craig, A. (1981). *Marriage dead or alive*. Dallas, TX: Spring Publications.

Modell, A. (1971). The origin of certain forms of pre-Oedipal guilt and the implications for a psychoanalytic theory of affects. *International Journal of Psycho-Analysis*. 52, 337-346.

Niederland, W. (1981). The survivor syndrome: Further observations and dimensions. *Journal of the American Psychoanalytic Association*, 29, 413-423.

Rheingold, J.C. (1964). *The fear of being a woman: a theory of maternal destructiveness*. New York: Grune & Stratton.

Wallerstein, J. & Blakeslee, S. (1995). *The good marriage*. Boston, New York: Houghton Mifflin Company.

Weiss, J. & Sampson, H. (1986). *The psychoanalytic process*. New York: The Guilford Press.

Weiss, J. (1993). *How psychotherapy works*. New York: The Guilford Press.

"I Sleep, But My Heart Stirs, Restless, and Dreams . . . ": The Mythology of Russian Jewish Immigrant Couples in Israel

Kris Jeter
Rita N. Gerasimova

Once upon a time, two itinerant scholars met at a roadhouse. Over coffee, they discussed their individual pilgrimages and soon discovered the similarities of their philosophies and work. They decided to cast their lots together, to ask the questions which restore wholeness.

These two new friends spoke with couples who had made the commitment to start their life anew in a strange land. To each couple, they posed questions about the stories of their lives, the image of homelands, the mythology of their immigrations. They had many delightful conversations and made numerous friends. Yet, their research questions remained unanswered. The boon of the hero's journey may not be readily predicted.

This story is true. In April 1992, the authors of this article, Rita N. Gerasimova and Kris Jeter, met over breakfast at the Youth Hostel in Beersheva, Israel. Gerasimova was functioning with a faculty exchange program from the University of Moscow, teaching English to Russian

---

Kris Jeter and Rita N. Gerasimova are both PhD's.

[Haworth co-indexing entry note]: "'I Sleep, But My Heart Stirs, Restless, and Dreams . . . ': The Mythology of Russian Jewish Immigrant Couples in Israel." Jeter, Kris, and Rita N. Gerasimova. Co-published simultaneously in *Journal of Couples Therapy* (The Haworth Press, Inc.) Vol. 7, No. 4, 1998, pp. 81-96; and: *Couples, Trauma, and Catastrophes* (ed: Barbara Jo Brothers) The Haworth Press, Inc., 1998, pp. 81-96. Single or multiple copies of this article are available for a fee from The Haworth Document Delivery Service [1-800-342-9678, 9:00 a.m. - 5:00 p.m. (EST). E-mail address: getinfo@haworthpressinc.com].

© 1998 by The Haworth Press, Inc. All rights reserved.

immigrant engineers at Ben Gurion University. Jeter was conducting various research projects in archetypal psychology. Gerasimova had been translator for a number of American psychologists on speaking tours in Russia and we both praised the effect of Carl Rogers and others on our personal and professional lives.

We talked of Israel's absorption of Russian immigrants. Gerasimova said that many recent immigrants lived in Caravans (mobile-homes) in a Beersheva suburb, so we drove to the central city's bus stop for the Caravans. Gerasimova asked if anyone who spoke Russian would accept a ride to direct us to the Caravans. A man and a woman offered to assist us. As we drove two miles to the Caravans, Gerasimova answered questions about conditions in the former U.S.S.R. when she left two months before.

We were invited to two homes, served coffee and home-made Russian drinks and foods. News spread quickly around the Caravans and other Russians gathered. Many wanted to meet the visiting Russian and American, share their story, hear of life at home and in the United States. Jeter was curious about the images and mythology that inspired these Russian couples to chose to immigrate to Israel. Gerasimova provided expert simultaneous translation.

Over the next two months we asked questions informally of couples and members of couples in the Caravans and at Ben Gurion University, attempting to determine the mythology underlying the decision to immigrate to Israel. We did not receive an answer, despite careful preparation of questions, the establishment of trust, the open two-way communication, the non-judgmental environment, the creativity, the definitions, and the examples.

Since then, we have wondered about the reasons why our respondents did not appear to associate their immigration and their homelands to Bible stories, fairy tales, folklore, images, or mythology. The experience of another scholar gave us an insight.

During this same time period, the spring of 1992, David Plante (1992) lectured at the Gorky Literary Institute in Moscow. Plante asked the learners what inspired their writing, especially "now, that they were free to write about whatever they wanted." After much silence, a learner answered, "The vision of Communism doomed us." Plante re-asked the question, "Don't you have any images, just images, that inspire you from what is happening now?" "What images?" was the response.

Later, a student said to Plante, "You were right, what you said to us. We must look for images, just images. But we cannot see them. We look, but we cannot now see them."

PREMISE OF THE STUDY

All beginnings are difficult.

–Midrash

Mobility, the pulling up of roots and planting them in another continent, requires that the couple be highly motivated. Often, concern over one's physical health and safety plus improvement of economic status are given reasons. Yet, underlying these apparent motives lies a deeper yearning based on the mythology of the spirit, the psychology of the soul. In spite of 75 years of state-focused ideology, a deep archetypal sleep, does not the "heart stir, restless, and dream . . ." (Falk, 1990)?

What age old images and stories remain to ignite couples to leave "Mother Russia," to start life anew in Israel, the 4,000 year old home of Mother Sarah and Father Abraham?

In this analytic essay, we analyze our initial subjective pilot study. We call upon the Muses in each of us to reflect and play with reasons for this almost total absence of stories embodying myths which guide everyday life. What follows is an explanation more from the heart than from interpretations of research data.

First, we discuss the demography of Jewish Russian couples historically in Russia and presently in Israel. We present historical reasons why our respondents may not have known or shared images and mythological motives for their immigration. We then suggest two ways in which images and mythology have survived. We conclude by offering an age-old Jewish folk story which may touch the souls and enlighten the spirits of Russian Jewish immigrant couples in Israel.

On 19 August 1991, the U.S.S.R. experienced an unsuccessful and nearly bloodless coup. Thus far, 15 provinces (Armenia, Azerbaijan, Belarus, Estonia, Georgia, Kazakhstan, Kyrgyzstan, Latvia, Lithuania, Moldava, Russian Federation, Tajikistan, Turkmenistan, Ukraine, Uzbekistan) have declared independence ("Name Changes in the Former Soviet Union," 1992 and "Soviet Union Frees Baltic Republics," 1991). Throughout this paper, we shall use the term "Russia" as a synonym for the former Russian Empire, the former U.S.S.R., and the contemporary independent states. "Russian Jews" will refer to Jews who have lived or presently live in this territory which includes Belorussia, Lithuania, and the Ukraine.

JEWISH COUPLES IN THE FORMER U.S.S.R. AND IN ISRAEL

Matchmaker, matchmaker, make me a match.

–*Fiddler on the Roof*

Historians are astonished by the persistence of the Jewish people to retain an identity, especially while in exile and the Diaspora, for four thousand years. Other cultures have died either because of refusal to assimilate or as a consequence of excessive assimilation. Indeed, in Russia, intermarriage has threatened the Jewish identity.

The 1926 census (Nove and Neweth, 1969, pages 134-135) for the U.S.S.R. indicates significant intermarriage. Twenty-five per cent of marriages involving at least one Jewish partner were between a Jewish husband and a non-Jewish wife. Seventeen per cent of such marriages were between a Jewish wife and a non-Jewish husband.

With the Bolshevik Revolution's extensive development of urbanization and occupations suited to industrialization, craft and trade, the livelihood of many rural Jews, was eliminated. People, especially young men, moved to the larger cities such as Kiev, Moscow, Odessa, and Petrograd. Jewish men would marry at an older age than non-Jewish men. Even so, the pool of potential Jewish wives did not equal the number of available Jewish men.

Mixed marriages were not as common in the rural areas to the West where Yiddish was the primary language. However, the survivors of the Nazi war crimes tended to be the Jews who had assimilated with the Russian culture. Thus, after World War II, intermarriage increased also in the rural areas.

In 1959, the Jewish population in the U.S.S.R. was over two million; thirty years later, it had shrunk to less than one and one half million. "The population decrease is caused by very low fertility rates, rising assimilation and intermarriage, a preference for non-Jewish national affiliation for the offspring of mixed marriages, and rapid and acute aging" (Greenwood, 1991, pages 218-219).

Indeed, in the Slavic Republics, in 1978, half of all Jewish men and 37% of all Jewish women were in a mixed marriage. During the next decade, these percentages rose over one per cent a year.

The latest statistics of the Ukraine indicates that 57% of Jewish women marry non-Jewish men. Only six per cent of their children consider themselves to be Jewish (Erlanger, 1992).

Jews have lived in Israel for four thousand years. For the past two thousand years, Israel has been ruled by non-Jews, and most Jews have lived in the Diaspora. It was not until 1948 that Israel once again became a Jewish state. Under the Law of Return, every Jew, plus first-and second-generation offspring of Jews with the members of their household, are granted the right to enter Israel and obtain citizenship upon request. The Jewish family is returning to the homeland. Some Jews believe that when every member of the Jewish family has returned, when the land of Israel is redeemed, the Messianic Age will dawn for the entire world.

Since 1989, the former Soviet Union has allowed Jews to leave Russia. Over 300,000 have immigrated to Israel. Both partners in eighty-nine per cent of the married couples are Jewish. Five per cent of the couples have a non-Jewish wife and a Jewish husband; 4.3 per cent have a Jewish wife and a non-Jewish husband. Almost 2 per cent of the couples are not themselves Jewish, for example those whose grandparents are Jewish. Thus, Russian couples choosing to immigrate to Israel tend to be less intermarried than the population remaining in the former U.S.S.R.

WHEN RIDING THE ROLLER COASTER OF HISTORY, WHAT IS A COUPLE TO BELIEVE?

Historically, Russian Jews have been riding a roller coaster of paradox. Couples, many intermarried, have had to survive unpredictable bi-polar realities. This has been true not only within their own marriage, but even more so as they attempt to hold on to the rails of the societal roller coaster.

Since the Partitions of Poland in 1772, 1793, and 1795, Jewish communities were under the political control of the Russian Empire instead of the Polish Commonwealth. Jewish communities were bound within "Pales of Settlement." Except for occasional expulsions and ever increasing taxes, life was stable. Jewish rituals and laws were exercised by the Beit Din (House of Judgement or Court of Law); relationships with the government were conducted by community leaders.

Then, Empress Catherine II attempted to fuse Jews to the Russian economy and legal system. Later, Alexander I attempted to attract Jews to participate in the Russian education system and farming colonies.

However, it was Nicholas I who treated Jews with unbelievable ferocity. Between 1850 and 1853, Nicholas I raised military conscription quotas and taxes to levels demographically unrealistic. For the next thirty years, over seventy thousand Jewish boys were drafted. In the military, they either were forced to convert or they died. Community leaders were forced to select the sacrificial conscripts, rapidly destroying the Jewish family and community infrastructure (Stanislawski, 1983, pages 183-186).

In the early nineteenth century, Russian Jews learned of the European Age of Enlightenment. By 1840, the Russian Jewish community was divided into two philosophies: the traditionalists and the enlightened. The traditionalists shielded themselves from change by deepening their beliefs and by the practice of the Orthodox religion. The enlightened sought to work with the government, sending their children to state schools for

Jewish children and attempting to integrate within the economic and social community. When Nicholas died, the enlightened had become a sanguine intelligentsia, committed to effecting modernity for the Jews of Russia (Stanislawski, 1983, pages 186-188).

In 1882, the May Laws were enforced, limiting the residence and employment of Jews. The 1881 and 1882 pogroms resulted in the death of many Jews (Grayzel, 1960, page 16). Many homeless survivors immigrated to countries with "streets of gold" in the Americas, Australia, and Europe and then communicated their experiences to their friends and families of their experiences. During the next two decades, two major groups of Russian Jews developed. The religious felt that life is Russia would be most authentic, suspected the ways of the emigrants, and immigrated only if conditions were unbearable and family members would absorb them in the new land. The second group were the socialists, well educated and aware of world events because of their communications with Russians who had already left of the nationalist movements. They believed that Russia would soon become democratic (Grayzel, 1960, page 61).

World War I was fought primarily in the Pale, the primary home of Jews in Russia. Alternately Germans and then Russians would befriend and then persecute Jews in the Pale. Jews, accused of being slackers, were actually the largest groups proportionately in all of the armies. Thus, Jews suffered extraordinary casualties in both civilian and military life (Grayzel, 1960, page 77).

Following World War I, the Czar was toppled by the democratic Kerensky government, which was quickly overturned by the Bolsheviks. In the Ukraine, systematically organized pogroms killed many Jews. Officially, the pogroms were not sanctioned, but, they were readily allowed (Grayzel, 1960, page 78).

The services of merchants, often Jews, were no longer required by Communists. Youth could learn to work in factories or on farms. Elders, however, assumed menial tasks and often starved (Nove and Newth, 1970, page 131). Meanwhile, religious education and practice, as well as use of the Hebrew language, were labeled counter-revolutionary. Thousands of Jews disobeyed these laws and were sent to prisons and Siberian work camps. Many died. Food and medical care were insufficient. Guards, at will, would often torture and kill prisoners. Despite the likelihood of this punishment, the Zionist youth movement flourished (Schechtman, 1970, pages 108-109).

On 14 May 1948, Israel proclaimed its statehood. The U.S.S.R. was the first country to acknowledge Israeli independence. The Kremlin allowed

Czechoslovakia to sell arms to Israel, which needed them to fight the War of Independence. Actually, this support was motivated by the Soviet desire to replace the British in the Middle East (Schechtman, 1970, pages 116-117).

In 1957, the U.S.S.R. invited internationals to participate in the International Youth Festival in Moscow. Two hundred Israeli delegates were eagerly welcomed by crowds of Russian Jews. After the Festival, thousands of Jews were accused of "fraternization" and fired from their jobs, arrested, and even sent to Siberian work camps (Schechtman, 1970, page 119).

Again and again, Russian Jews have been riding a roller coaster of paradox. Throughout the twentieth century, couples have been faced with choosing to cast their lot with the traditionalists or enlightened, the Orthodox or intelligentsia, the democrats or socialists, the Germans or Russians, silence or Siberian work camps. Bi-polar realities emanated from a capricious, inhuman, narrow, onerous, and paternalistic government for Jews and Gentiles alike.

WHO IDENTIFIES JEWS?

One Russian Jew told of his childhood. His parents died when he was very young and he was reared by a Christian relative. The children at school called him a "Jew." He had no idea what a Jew was and so researched the topic in the library. He spent his youth reading about the identity thrust him by his neighbors. Today, he is a University librarian and scholar, assisting other Jews in search of their identity.

Aleksandr A. Shalyen, director of the Babi Yar Center in Kiev, told Steven Erlanger (1992), "They started to beat the Jewishness out of Jews a long time ago, under the czars." Then, Communism sought systematically to erase the cultural and religious identity of Jews. Practices were forbidden and information was limited. "The last of the culture-bearers were executed . . ."

Yiddish writers of the nineteenth century had written of the glory of the Jewish soul and spirit. With the revolution, Russian Jewish writers now yielded to Communism. The new Russia would be fashioned by Jews. Religion, Hebrew, Yiddish, and Zionism were not needed. Their style was cynical, obscure, realistic, and Western. However, historical fiction was very popular and did recollect the dauntless resolution of the Jews.

In 1948, almost every Jewish author was transported to a Siberian work camp. The Yiddish publishing house was closed. A year later, the Jewish State Theatre was shut down.

Without literature, schools, synagogues, and rabbis, the Jewish community was to die. In 1959, the government responded to the world's criticism and allowed the Hebrew prayer book and a small volume of Shalom Aleichem stories to be published (Korey, 1970, pages 85-87). In 1961, a Yiddish literary magazine, *Sovietish Heymland,* was inaugurated. Even the *Sovietish Heymland* publishes anti-Israel and anti-Jewish writings (Levine, 1987, page 127). The following year, a Yiddish repertory company started touring the country. As the Russian language replaced the use of Yiddish, intermarriage increased (Korey, 1970, pages 85-87).

The official publication of anti-religious propaganda, macabre stories illustrated with hooked nosed caricatures, provoked anti-Semitic acts (Schapiro, 1970, pages 6-7). Money was said to be the Jewish deity. Because Jews considered themselves to be the chosen people, they were portrayed as hating non-Jews. Zionism meant loyalty to Israel, not Russia (Rothenberg, 1970, page 177).

> . . . Hitler and Stalin both won their wars against the Jews. They did not extirpate every last Jew, but in a way accomplished something almost as historic: they displaced a millennium of vibrant European Jewish civilization with a grotesquely malformed version of it. Where Hitler had reduced a thriving culture to pictures of skeletons and piles of corpses, Stalin allowed most Jews to live, but only after he had beat their Jewish brains out by purging Jewish intellectuals. With their writers and cultural figures murdered, their literature and art outlawed and all Jewish religious learning banned, two generations of Jews grew up defining their Jewishness on Stalin's terms alone. (Young, 1982, page 13)

After the Six Day War in 1967, anti-Zionist and anti-Israel news articles increased in radio and in print (Katz, 1970, pages 334-336). Israeli radio broadcasts in Russian beamed to the Soviet Union were jammed. During the 1970s, the interference with the radio waves increased (Nudel, 1989, page 220). With the recent break up of the Soviet Union into independent states and increased economic woes, a scapegoat has been required and anti-Semitism has dramatically increased (Wistrich, 1990).

Despite the Soviet strategies to destroy Judaism, it somehow survived in Russia. Elie Wiesel (1965, pages 68-69), on a visit to Russia during the High Holy Days in 1965, asked Jews, " 'Who is a Jew? What is Judaism? What makes you a Jew?' They shrugged their shoulders . . . They are Jews, and that is that; the rest is unimportant. A Jew is one who feels himself [or herself] a Jew."

What are the images of Judaism that stir the hearts of Russian Jewish

couples who feel themselves to be Jewish? What ancient Jewish mythology is being repeated today by Russian Jewish couples who choose to go to
live in Israel?

IMAGE AND MYTHOLOGY

Where people truly wish to go,
there their feet will manage to take them.

-The Talmud

The image is the way in which one senses–hears, sees, smells, tastes,
touches–life. Imaging is the act of sensing and perceiving. The image–the
art, music, and poetry of the mind–speaks to the soul and spirit.

Mythology is a collection of images and the fountainhead of an individual's and a community's belief system. Mythology is imbedded in
culture and is a deep seated rationale for behavior. The word mythology
is derived from the Greek, *muthos*, which means word or speech.
Mythology is the embodiment of the divine in words; it chronicles for a
social community the origins, foundation, intentions, and essence of the
world. Mythology is the paradigm for action, enlightenment, and sagac-
ity for the cultural group. Mythology may be conveyed by action, art,
location, or word.

Mythology gives each social group a sense of ancestry, identity, pride,
purpose, strength, and uniqueness. Embroiled in the myth are realities
which are separated into polar opposites: the intellectual and the illogical,
the practical and the idealistic, the physical and the emotional, the material
and the celestial, the mortal and the divine, Christian and Jewish. Within
the context of the story, these varied realties are presented as a unified
whole. The listener's mind set is challenged to recognize the harmony of
the universe despite, and in fact, because of the multiplicity of options.
Anything is possible within the orchestration of seemingly contradictory
ways of being.

Most Jews go to Israel to fulfill four-thousand-year-old dreams for
home, the "Land of Milk and Honey." Jerusalem is remembered as the
capitol of King David who "lives now and forever more."

Are Russian Jews immigrating to Israel only because of surface reasons? Some have said that Russian Jews are like the "proverbial rats
leaving a sinking ship," departing the former U.S.S.R. where 80 per cent
of the population lives below the poverty level (Cohen, 1992). As in most
migrations in the world's history, parents leave with the knowledge that
adjustment may be difficult for them, but that life will be better for the

children. In Israel, parents can feel assured that their children can marry Jews.

Ida Nudel (1989, page 220) has written that Russian Jews who immigrate to Israel are emotionally sensitive and expressive social activists. They are educated, especially in the sciences, and to "succeed in the hostile Russian society, developed a high self-esteem." They enjoy telling stories of the hardships of their immigration.

But, what are the imaginal and mythological motives for migration? Can they be identified?

Admittedly, Russian immigrants to Israel are living under tensions common to mobile, immigrant families. It is stressful to leave a home to forge a life in an unknown culture with a different climate, economy, government, language, social structure, and religion. The democratic freedom for an individual to make choices can be overwhelming. Meanwhile, the difficulty for Russians to learn to live in today's democratic Russia instead of Communism has been addressed by Economic Minister Andrei Nechayev, "the main obstacle we face is the Soviet mentality: the willingness of people to continue to live badly as long as they are all equal and do not have to work very hard. To change this mentality is proving very difficult" (Dobbs, 1992, page 18).

Moreover, American and Israeli society is openly analyzed, discussed, and debated. Russian society is very isolated and covert. Americans and Israelis assume that if a person knows something, it will be told and will be part of the common knowledge. Russians under Communism learned for survival to be secretive (Glazer, 1992; Molinari, 1992). In Communist Russia, has history been buried so deep that it is the popular mythology of the day?

Fear has been predominant in Czarist and Communist Russia. There is no reason for Russians to trust anyone and even less reason for Russian Jews to trust anyone. Depression has been a common reaction to fear (Molinari, 1992). Therapist Barbara Glazer, for example, never heard any stories from either of her Russian grandparents. Glazer believes that their life was so difficult, it was better to forget the past completely and start anew. Even today, "everything in Russia is in flux. The trauma of Communism, still inadequately appreciated in the West (in no small measure thanks to years of soothing misinformation dispensed by fellow-travelers and 'value-free' social scientists), had created in the majority of the population, especially among the better educated, a revulsion against the past" (Pipes, 1992).

The images and mythology do emerge, however, out of the stress of migration and generations of isolation, secrets, fear, and depression. Courageous will power, creative expression, and Jewish identity have triumphed over seventy-five years of state focused ideology. Indeed, despite the deep archetypal sleep, the "heart stirs, restless, and dreams . . . " (Falk, 1990) of Israel, the land of the family of Jews.

TRADITION

Recent research (Nellhaus, 1992; Patai, 1983; Patai, 1983) on crypto-Jews of Spanish descent who have lived in Mexico and southwestern United States for 500 years has provided valuable insights. Crypto-Jews are descendants of *conversos*, Spanish Jews who openly converted to Catholicism and secretly practised Judaism. Traditions such as cleaning house on Friday, not working on Saturday, and celebration of *El Dia Grande* in early autumn have survived, very often without conscious, verbal rationale.

Likewise, a Russian couple spoke of sneaking into the synagogue to look at the Jewish calendar to discover when to fast and when to feast. The actual family traditional celebrations are vital, living links to Judaism for both the Jews of Mexico and southwestern United States whose ancestors lived through the Inquisition and the Jews of Russia who persevered Czars and Communism. The images provided to the taste buds have survived generations of public policies to suppress cultural identity. For instance, round challah bread topped with sweets has been baked each year for the uniquely Russian celebration of Purim.

For Russian Jews, Jewish cuisine has especially been the proverbial straw clutched by the drowning person. For generations, recipes were transmitted from mother to daughter. Only in 1989, was the first Jewish cookbook available for purchase in the Soviet Union. Tschizova (1991) has proposed that the varied and numerous national cuisines in the U.S.S.R. were catalysts for liberating expressions of pride in ancestral heritage and even facilitated public acknowledgement of minority cultures. Ethnic cuisines had an everyday life character, rather than sacred character. They gave minority groups a chance to feel closer to their particular ethnic culture and identity without experiencing fear of repression. Moreover, it was an opportunity for Gentiles to understand that "these people are Jews; they are different."

HUMOR

Humor was the primary story telling mode utilized by Russian immigrant couples. Depression, fear, pain, and secrecy can be addressed under the mask of humor. Below are two jokes told to us.

Joke 1: *Immigration is a question of lines. You either stand in lines in Russia to buy food or you stand in lines in Israel to get a job!*

Joke 2: *Female: In 1990, I visited friends in Israel and felt so at home, I decided to immigrate.*
Male: Of course you would feel at home in Israel. Everyone speaks Russian!

These jokes are reminiscent of humorous folklore about the matchmaker or *shadchan* (Ausubel, 1948, page 414).

> *A shadchan speaks to a man of an available woman, suggesting that they marry. The man says, "Why would I want a blind wife?" The shadchan replies, "A blind wife allows you do what you want." The man says, "She is mute." "So, you will never hear a complaint." "She is deaf." "So, she will never hear you complain." "She is lame." "So, she cannot follow you when you chase other women." "She is hunchbacked." "I do not like your finickiness. Can you not accept one flaw in your future wife?"*

THE HEART'S DREAM

Some Russian immigrant couples in Israel may feel as if they have arrived in Israel because of their naive acceptance of the advice of an archetypal *shadchan*. The stresses of moving, learning a new language, looking for employment, and adapting to a new culture either strengthen or loosen the bonds of a couple. Over one century of waves of immigration have shown Israelis that absorption does take place. Social workers predict that within five years it is difficult to tell a Russian immigrant from a native born *sabra* (Guttman, 1992). Schooling and military service integrate the young. Intermarriage interweaves Jewish families of different cultures.

In conclusion, images and mythology can serve as a framework in which individuals and couples place experiences. Life can be viewed archetypally and its meaning ennobled. The repetition of age-old traditions, as well as the spontaneous telling of jokes, are just two of a variety of ways to express image and live once again in potent mythic time and space. The 75-year sleep was not in vain, but rather a crucible for the dreams of the future and the stirrings of the heart. The Hebrew Bible (I Kings 10: 1-13) tells the story of the Queen of Sheba's visit with King Solomon. Many subsequent ancient mythological folk tales have suggested that the Queen of Sheba and King Solomon had romantic interests in each other and became a couple. Below is one which may serve as a story of hope for immigrant couples (Aububel, 1948, pages 480-487; Noy, 1964, page 174; Patai, 1981, pages 70-73).

Once upon a time, King Solomon heard from travelers about the intelligent, gracious, and beautiful ruler, The Queen of Sheba. The King sent the Queen an official invitation to visit him in Jerusalem. The Queen of Sheba rushed to be with him, completing the seven year journey in just three years. Upon meeting, they felt as if they had known each other all of their lives and their relationship blossomed. As a couple, they challenged, benefited, grew, and gloried in each other's wisdom.

However, King Solomon found himself suffering from bouts of depression. The Queen of Sheba presented him with a ring upon which was engraved "Gamzu ya'avor" (This too will pass.) Whenever the King would feel depressed, he would simply touch the ring, gaze upon its message, and the depression would be transmuted into courage to greet life's problems as opportunities.

The Queen of Sheba and King Solomon continued to live, according to their heart's desire, responding to life's crescendos and nadirs as if in the center of a wheel, confident that "This too will pass." They had learned that life on the edge of a wheel is a very bumpy ride. We, their humble children, are blessed to have such notable parents as our ancestors and such a hallowed path to follow.

REFERENCES

Ausubel, Nathan, editor (1948). *A treasury of Jewish folklore.* New York, NY: Crown Publishers.

Billington, James H. (1966). *The icon and the axe.* New York NY: Knopf.

Billington, James H. (1992). *Russia transformed: breakthrough to hope, Moscow, August 1991.* Toronto, Canada: Free Press.

Brothers, Barbara Jo (6 June 1992). Personal communication. Port Jervis, NY.

Campbell, Joseph with Bill Moyers (1988). *The power of myth.* New York, NY: Doubleday.

Cohen, Stephen (19 August 1992). *CBS news up to the minute.*

Dobbs, Michael (24-30 August 1992). "Russia, one year later: arguing every step of the way." *The Washington Post,* 9: 43, 16-18.

Dubnow, Simon (1916-1920). *The history of Jews in Russia and Poland.* Philadelphia, PA: Jewish Publication Society.

Erlanger, Steven (27 August 1992). "As Ukraine loses Jews, the Jews lose a tradition." *The New York Times,* A3.

Falk, Marcia, Translator (1990). *The Song of Songs: love lyrics from the Bible.* San Francisco CA: Harper, Poem 19.

Frankel, Jonathan (1981). *Prophecy and politics: socialism, nationalism and the Russian Jews, 1862-7917.* Cambridge, England: Cambridge University Press.

Gitelman, Zvi Y. (1988). *A century of ambivalence: The Jews of Russia and the Soviet Union, 1881 to the present.* New York, NY: Schocken Books.

Gitelman, Zvi Y (1972). *Jewish nationality and Soviet politics.* Princeton, NJ: Princeton University.

Glazer, Barbara (6 June 1992). Private Communication. Port Jervis, NY.

Grayzel, Solomon (1960). *A history of the contemporary Jews from 7900 to present.* New York, NY: Meridian Books.

Greenwood, Naftali, editor (1992). "Aliya 1991: back from the USSR." *Israel Yearbook and Almanac 1991/2.* Volume 46. Jerusalem, Israel: IBRT Translation/Documentation Ltd.

Guttman, David (1 June 1992). Private communication. Haifa, Israel.

Heer, Friedrich (1970). *God's first love.* New York, NY: Weybright and Talley.

Hillman, James (1983). *Archetypal psychology.* Dallas, TX: Spring Publications, Inc.

Hoffman, Charles (1992). *Gray Dawn: The Jews of Eastern Europe in the Post-Communist Era.* New York, NY: Aaron Asher Books/Harper Collings Publishers.

The holy Bible (_). King James Version. New York, NY: American Bible Society.

Jeter, Kris (1990). "Kings and Scapegoats in Twentieth Century Families and Corporations." *Marriage and Family Review: Corporations, Businesses and Families* 15: 3/4, 225-242.

Jung, Carl G. (1969). *The archetypes and the collective unconscious.* Second edition. R.F.C. Hull, translator. Princeton, NJ: Princeton University Press.

Katz, Zev (1969). "After the Six-Day War." *The Jews in Soviet Russia since 1917.* Kochan, Lionel, editor. London, England: Oxford University Press, 321-336.

Kochan, Lionel, editor (1969). *The Jews in Soviet Russia since 1917.* London, England: Oxford University Press.

Korey, W. (1969). "The legal position of Soviet Jewry: A historical enquiry." *The Jews in Soviet Russia since 1917.* Kochan, Lionel, editor. London, England: Oxford University Press, 76-98.

Kutnick, Jerry (9 August 1992). "Zionism and the Messianic idea." *The Jewish Idea of the Messiah.* Philadelphia, PA: Congregation Mikveh Israel.

Levin, Nora (1987). "The Problematic of *Sovetish Heymland.*" *Community and Culture: Essays in Jewish Studies in Honor of the 90th Anniversary of Gratz College.* Nahum M. Waldman, editor. Philadelphia, PA: Gratz College, Seth Press.

Molinari, Margaret (6 June 1992). Personal Communication. Port Jervis, NY.

"Name changes in the former Soviet Union" (1-5 January 1992). *Facts on File* 52: 2667, 1.

Nellhaus, Arlynn (29 May 1992). "Unraveling the secrets of the Crypto-Jews." *The Jerusalem Post Magazine* 12, 15.

Nove, Alec and J.A. Newth (1969). "The Jewish population: Demographic Trends and Occupational Patterns." *The Jews in Soviet Russia since 1917.* Kochan, Lionel, editor. London, England: Oxford University Press, 125-158.

Noy, Dov, editor (1963). *Folktales of Israel.* Chicago, IL: The University of Chicago Press, 174.

Nudel, Ida (1989). "Soviet Jewry: time is running out." *Israel Yearbook 1989.* Volume 44. Tel Aviv, Israel: Israel Yearbook Publications, Ltd.

Patai, Raphael (1981). *Gates to the old city: a book of Jewish legends.* Detroit MI: Wayne State University Press.

Patai, Raphael (1983). "The Jewish Indians of Mexico." *On Jewish Folklore.* Detroit MI: Wayne State University Press, 447-475.

Patai, Raphael (1983). "Venta Prieta revisited." *On Jewish Folklore.* Detroit MI: Wayne State University Press, 476-492.

Pipes, Richard (24-30 August 1992). "Communism on trail: this time in Moscow." *The Washington Post National Weekly Edition,* 9: 43, 24.

Prital, David (1989). "Jews in the Soviet Union." *Israel Yearbook 1989.* Volume 44. Tel Aviv, Israel: Israel Yearbook Publications, Ltd.

Prital, David (1988). "Soviet Jewish immigration to Israel in 1987." *Israel Yearbook 1988.* Volume 43. Tel Aviv, Israel: Israel Yearbook Publications, Ltd.

Plante, David (19 July 1992). "We in Russia have had enough of ideas." *The New York Times Book Review,* 1, 33, 34, 35.

Rafael, Gideon (1988). "Time for restructuring." *Israel Yearbook 1988.* Volume 43. Tel Aviv, Israel: Israel Yearbook Publications, Ltd.

Rogger, Hans. "Russian ministers and the Jewish question, 1881-1917." *California Slavic Studies* 8 (1975) 15-76.

Rothenberg, J. (1969). "Jewish religion in the Soviet Union." *The Jews in Soviet Russia since 1917.* Kochan, Lionel. editor. London, England: Oxford University Press, 159-187.

Ruether, Rosemary (1974). *Faith and fratricide: the theological roots of antisemitism.* New York, NY: Seabury Press.

Schapiro, L. (1969). "Introduction." *The Jews in Soviet Russia since 1917.* Kochan, Lionel, editor. London, England: Oxford University Press, 1-14.

Schechtman, J.B. (1969). "The U.S.S.R., Zionism, and Israel." *The Jews In Soviet Russia since 1917.* Kochan, Lionel, editor. London, England: Oxford University Press, 99-124.

Stanislawski, Michael (1983). *Tsar Nicholas I and the Jews.* Philadelphia, PA. Jewish Publication Society of America.

Sheynin, Hayim Y. (22 July 1992). Private Communication. Philadelphia, PA: Gratz College.

"Soviet Union frees Baltic Republics: Estonia, Latvia, Lithuania" (12 September 1991). *Facts on File,* 51: 2651, 669.

Tschizova, Ludmila (1991). "The Museum Under the Conditions of International Conflicts: Materials of the All-Union Scientific Conference." *International*

Problems of Conflict: Searching for Resolving. U.S.S.R.: Bishkek. (Russian language.)

Tumashkova, Natasha (8 December 1991). "What is Woman? What is Man? Some answers in fairy tales." Port Jervis, NY. Personal Communication.

Tzion, Ben (3 May 1970). "The Jewish question in the Soviet Union." *The New York Times Magazine. New York Times.*

Walker, Martin (1986). *The Waking Giant.* London, England: Joseph.

Wiesel, Elie (1987). *The Jews of silence: A personal report on Soviet Jewry.* Neal Kozodoy, translator. New York, NY: Schocken Books.

Wistrich, Robert S. (1992). *Antisemitism: the longest hatred.* New York, NY: Pantheon.

Young, James E. (6 September 1992). "Living at the Scene of the Crime." *The New York Times Book Review*, 12-13.

Index

Anxiety
    child snatching and, 39
    Holocaust survivor guilt and, 70

Boundary clarification, in elective
    pediatric amputation, 50-51

Case examples
    of elective pediatric amputation
      (CPT), 51,53-57
    of envious family members, 77-78
    of families of origin issues, 53
    of gender issues, during ill infant
      care, 56-57
    of honoring trauma, 9-10
    of mothers, distancing from,
      73-75
    of naming the trauma, power of,
      8-9
    of parental abduction, 40-45
    of parental miscommunication, 37
    of professional reaction, 54
    of self-infliction of punishment,
      72
    of siblings of disabled children,
      55-56
    of survivor guilt, 71-78
    of "transference test" of therapist,
      75-76
    of traumatized couples therapy,
      11-17
    of withholding responses, 73-74
Catastrophic illness, intimacy and
    "best things" concept and, 67
    coping resources and, 64
    "death"/"rebirth" process and,
      66-67

HDC/BMT process and, 66
healing circles and, 65-66
intimacy levels and, 63
summary regarding, 63
time, preciousness of, 66
ways of relating and, 67
Child snatching. *See* Parental
    abduction
Congenital pseudarthrosis of the tibia
    (CPT).
    See Elective pediatric amputation
Couples therapy. *See* Traumatized
    couples therapy
CPT (congenital pseudarthrosis of
    the tibia).
    See Elective pediatric amputation
Cupp, Penny, 63

Death of a child, intimacy therapy
    for
    "becoming one disciplines" stage
      of, 31-33
    case scenario of, 23
    comfort, giving and receiving of,
      29,33
    communication, interruption in,
      20-21,26,31
    confession and forgiveness and,
      26,28-29,33
    emotional responding stage of,
      22-23,27-29,28*fig.*,33
    families of origin reflection stage
      of, 25,30-31
    fear of losing wife and, 21
    foci of, 33-34
    guilt and, 29
    helplessness, husband's sense of,
      20
    intergenerational issues and, 23

© 1998 by The Haworth Press, Inc. All rights reserved.

Printed and bound by CPI Group (UK) Ltd, Croydon, CR0 4YY

17/10/2024

01775686-0003